AMBULATORY TREATMENT OF VENOUS DISEASE:

An Illustrative Guide

AMBULATORY TREATMENT OF VENOUS DISEASE:
An Illustrative Guide

MITCHEL P. GOLDMAN, M.D.
JOHN J. BERGAN, M.D.

With 217 illustrations, 158 in 4-color

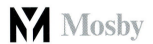 Mosby

St. Louis Baltimore Boston Carlsbad Chicago Naples New York Philadelphia Portland
London Madrid Mexico City Singapore Sydney Tokyo Toronto Wiesbaden

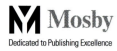
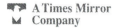

Publisher: Anne S. Patterson
Editor: Susie Baxter
Developmental Editor: Ellen Baker Geisel
Project Manager: Deborah Vogel
Production Manager: Karen Allman
Designer: A-R Editions, Inc.

Printed in the United States of America

Composition by A-R Editions, Inc.
Printing/Binding by Walsworth Press, Inc.

Mosby-Year Book, Inc.
11830 Westline Industrial Drive
St. Louis, Missouri 64146

International Standard Book Number 0–8151–3758–3

96 97 98 99 / 9 8 7 6 5 4 3 2 1

CONTRIBUTORS

John J. Bergan, M.D., F.A.C.S.
Clinical Professor of Surgery
University of California, San Diego;
Clinical Professor of Surgery
Uniformed Services University of the Health Sciences
Bethesda, Maryland;
Professor of Surgery
Loma Linda University Medical Center
Loma Linda, California

Ken P. Biegeleisen, M.D., F.A.C.A.
New York, New York

Simon G. Darke, M.S., F.R.C.S.
Lecturer
Southampton University;
Consultant Surgeon
Department of Vascular Surgery
Royal Bournemouth Hospital
Poole, Dorset, England

Bo Eklof, M.D., Ph.D.
Clinical Professor of Surgery
University of Hawaii
John A. Burns School of Medicine;
Vascular Surgeon
Straub Clinic and Hospital
Honolulu, Hawaii

Vin Frederic, M.D.
Chief of Phlebology
Notre Dame de Bon Secours Hospital
Paris, France

Helane S. Fronek, M.D.
Instructor in Medicine
University of California, San Diego
San Diego Medical School
San Diego, California;
Director, Varicose Vein Clinic
Division of Cardiothoracic and Vascular Surgery
Scripps Clinic and Research Foundation
LaJolla, California

Mihael Georgiev, M.D.
Rome, Italy

Mitchel P. Goldman, M.D.
Assistant Clinical Professor
Division of Dermatology
Department of Medicine
University of California, San Diego
San Diego, California

Mary Henry, M.D.
Lecturer
Dublin University and
The Royal College of Surgeons;
Medical Practitioner
The Varicose Vein Clinic
The Adelaide and Rotunda Hospitals
Dublin, Ireland

Robert L. Kistner, M.D.
Clinical Professor of Surgery
University of Hawaii
John A. Burns School of Medicine;
Vascular Surgeon
Straub Clinic and Hospital
Honolulu, Hawaii

H.A. Martino Neumann, M.D., Ph.D.
Professor and Chairman
Department of Dermatology
Academic Hospital Maastricht;
Department of Dermatology
Rijksuniversiteit Limburg
Maastricht, The Netherlands

Hugo Partsch, M.D.
Department of Dermatology
Wilhelminen Hospital
Vienna, Austria

John R. Pfeifer, M.D., F.A.C.S.
Associate Clinical Professor of Surgery
Wayne State University
Detroit, Michigan;
Director, Surgical Research
Department of Surgery
Providence Hospital
Southfield, Michigan

Pauline Raymond-Martimbeau, M.D.
Dallas Noninvasive Vascular
Laboratory
Dallas, Texas

Neil Sadick, M.D.
Clinical Assistant Professor
Department of Dermatology
Cornell University Medical College;
Attending Physician
Department of Dermatology
New York Hospital
New York, New York

Michel Schadeck, M.D.
St. Georges, France

Joseph G. Sladen, M.D., F.R.C.S.(S)
Clinical Professor
Department of Vascular Surgery
University of British Columbia;
Department of Vascular Surgery
St. Paul's Hosptial
Vancouver, British Columbia, Canada

George M. Somjen, M.D., M.S., F.R.A.C.S., F.R.C.S.(Ed)
Vascular Surgeon
The Vascular Centre
Mornington Peninsula Hospital
Frankston, Australia

Richard J. Tazelaar, M.D.
Department of Dermatology
Algemeen Ziekenhuis De Tjongerschans
Heerenveen, The Netherlands

Paul K. Thibault, M.B.
Director, Central Vein and Laser Clinic
Newcastle, New South Wales, Australia

Paul S. van Bemmelen, M.D.
Clinical Assistant Professor
Department of Surgery
State University of New York at
Stony Brook
Stony Brook, New York;
Attending Surgeon
John T. Mather Memorial Hospital
St. Charles Hospital
Port Jefferson, New York

Margaret A. Weiss, M.D.
Assistant Professor of Dermatology
Johns Hopkins University School of Medicine
Baltimore, Maryland

Robert A. Weiss, M.D.
Assistant Professor of Dermatology
Johns Hopkins University School of Medicine
Baltimore, Maryland

Preface

Treatment of venous dysfunction is returning to the medical scene. Evidence for this is the increasing number of publications in referenced journals, the strengthening and enlargement of the English-language journal, *Phlebology,* and in the development of teaching programs within academic institutions. Prior to World War II, and before the modern era of arterial reconstructive surgery, treatment of venous disease was the province of surgeons, and teaching was regularly performed. Surgery was done in-hospital, and patients remained bedfast or with limited ambulation for many days.

Now, as treatment of venous dysfunction returns, it does so in an entirely different setting. Virtually all care is now done on an outpatient basis. Dermatologists and some internists have a vital interest in care of venous problems. Because of this, the editors felt that a collection of methods employed by prominent workers in this field would be a valuable teaching and learning tool.

Treatment of the various aspects of venous insufficiency is not codified. Trends toward standardization emerge, but many differing viewpoints hold equal status. The casual reader of this book will see that conflicting points of view are expressed here. This may be disturbing to some who would like to have specific instructions on care of particular problems. But treatment of venous disease is not cookbook therapy. It cannot be charted by decision trees.

The editors realize that there are many ways to achieve the ultimate ends of improving venous function, decreasing patient morbidity, and bettering the lives of patients with venous insufficiency. The editors actually disagree with some of the viewpoints that are expressed in the following pages. However, they understand that the final sermon has not come down from the mount, and the last laws have not been set down to be displayed for all time.

Because evaluation and treatment of venous dysfunction falls into particular categories, this volume is so divided. The section on evaluation emphasizes noninvasive techniques in general and ultrasound in particular. The chapters on treatment of telangiectasias display many different thoughts, the sum of which will undoubtedly improve individual patient care in a number of clinics. Much wisdom is shown in the experiences described.

Treating large veins by injection occupies a large portion of this book, and an underlying theme of careful sclerotherapy and effective compression runs through these chapters. Finally, the section on surgical alternatives to sclerotherapy contains much new information. It will be evident to readers of this portion of the book that principles underlying such surgery are sound, but techniques used to achieve these vary greatly.

It is the earnest hope of the editors that this volume will be useful, that care of patients with venous dysfunction will improve, and that a greater number of patients will benefit from lessons learned here.

Mitchel P. Goldman
John J. Bergan
La Jolla, California

Contents

IV. SURGICAL ALTERNATIVES TO SCLEROTHERAPY

Part I

Evaluation

1

EVALUATION OF THE PATIENT WITH TELANGIECTASES

Paul K. Thibault

The term telangiectasia refers to visible cutaneous vessels measuring 0.1 to 1 mm in diameter.[1] When lower limb cutaneous vessels are dilated greater than 1 mm in diameter they are referred to as venulectases.[2,3] Frequently described as "spider," "sunburst" or "starburst veins," the presence of telangiectases and venulectases is generally regarded as a cosmetic condition which results the physician's tendency to simplify his or her evaluation and diagnosis and ignore subtle signs that may indicate a more extensive pathology. In the majority of patients the presence of telangiectatic leg veins is a manifestation of localized or diffuse subcutaneous venous dilation[2-7] (Fig. 1-1).

Initially lower limb telangiectases appear as faintly erythematous lines, but with time they become progressively more dilated, tortuous, elevated above the skin surface and blue. Although the initial presentation would indicate a cutaneous disorder, it is likely that the primary pathophysiology occurs in the subcutaneous blue reticular veins which either drain to saphenous branches or directly to the deep system via perforating veins[8,9] (Fig. 1-2).

The initial step in evaluating the patient with lower limb telangiectasia is a directed history. Unattractive or disfiguring visual appearance is the most common symptom of patients with telangiectases. However, mild to moderate pain is a well-recognized symptom.[2] The most common physical symptoms are dull, generalized aching particularly after prolonged standing, pain over a localized area of telangiectasia, throbbing pain on the lateral aspect of the leg, night cramps and restless legs. These symptoms may be aggravated by menstruation and warmer weather and relieved by activities such as walking.

Although genetic predisposition is the most important etiological factor in telangiectasia development, hormonal influences of estrogen and progesterone result in females being predominantly affected.[10] Therefore, essential information obtained in the history will include family history, age of onset, aggravation by past pregnancies, and past and present use of exogenous estrogen and progesterone for contraception or hormonal replacement. It is important to note physical symptoms of pain and whether the primary symptom is cosmetic because this can significantly influence patient expectations regarding treatment outcomes and consequently affect treatment decisions. Past history should include history of bleeding from telangiectases, episodes of superficial thrombophlebitis, major limb trauma, deep venous thrombosis, and previous treatment including surgery and sclerotherapy.

Clinical examination of the lower limbs commences with the patient standing on a platform in front of the physician. Good lighting is essential for a systematic inspection of each aspect of the leg from the groin to the toes. The patterns of telangiectases and their relationships to underlying reticular and varicose veins must be noted. Using duplex ultrasound examination, Thibault and associates[11] found that approximately 25% of patients with lower limb telangiectases have some degree of incompetence in the long or short saphenous systems. Therefore, careful palpation to detect these sources of reflux is necessary. If the associated reticular veins and branch varices are not easily detected when the patient is standing, they may become more obvious if the physician examines the supine patient under ample overhead fluorescent lighting.

To complete the clinical evaluation, photographs should be taken of each aspect of the leg affected by telangiectases. This step is essential to assess progress during treatment and to clarify whether adverse sequelae

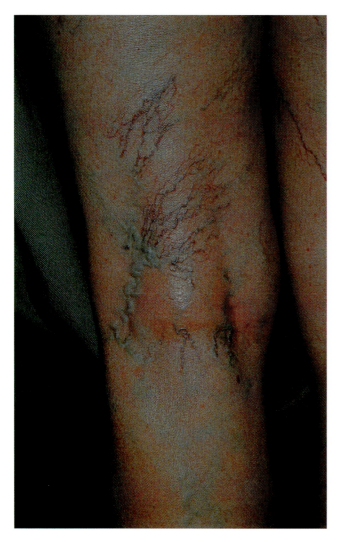

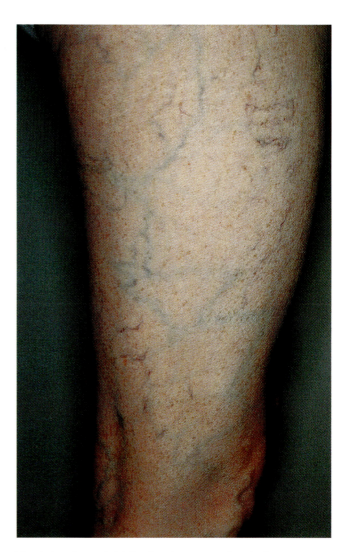

Fig. 1-1. Obvious association between telangiectases, venulectases, and subcutaneous varices on the posterior aspect of the leg of a 55-year-old woman. In most cases the association is more subtle.

Fig. 1-2. Lateral thigh telangiectases and reticular veins in a 53-year-old woman. Note the blue subcutaneous reticular veins drain toward the popliteal fossa and to varicose veins on the lateral aspect of the patella. Reflux in the reticular veins can be demonstrated by either bidirectional Doppler or duplex examination.

(such as telangiectatic matting) have occurred as a result of treatment.[3]

Following the physical examination, the experienced physician will be able to determine whether further evaluation with Doppler, photoplethysmography, or duplex examination is required to confirm the presence and extent of axial vein reflux, perforating vein, or junctional reflux and deep venous insufficiency. The decision regarding further evaluation will depend largely on the patterns of telangiectases detected on clinical examination.

PATTERNS OF LOWER LIMB TELANGIECTASES AND THEIR CLINICAL SIGNIFICANCE

Essential Progressive Telangiectasia

Essential progressive telangiectasia is a relatively rare, generalized acquired condition that develops independently of varices in the subcutaneous veins and is not related to other systemic disease.[12] Owing to hydrostatic pressures, the lower limbs and in particular the calves and feet are more extensively involved than other parts of the body (Fig. 1-3). The lesions appear as

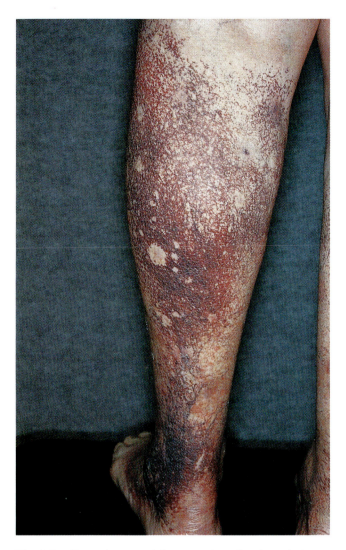

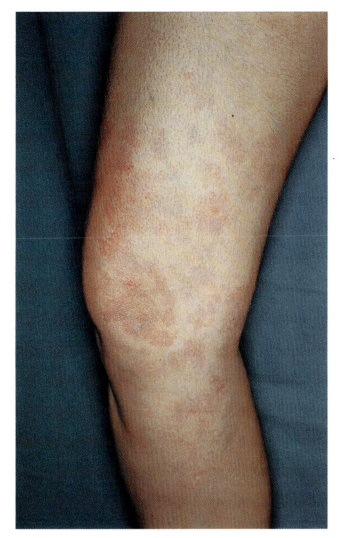

Fig. 1-3. Extensive essential progressive telangiectasia in a 71-year-old woman. This asymptomatic condition had been present for many years and was slowly progressive. The hypopigmented areas on the midcalf were the result of previous cryotherapy to actinic keratoses.

Fig. 1-4. Cutis marmorata telangiectatica congenita in an 18-year-old female. The condition had faded in appearance since birth and can be differentiated from the Klippel-Trénauney-Weber syndrome by absence of underlying varicose veins, deep venous abnormalities, arteriovenous anastomoses, and hypertrophy of soft tissue and bone.

blue or bright red telangiectases that refill rapidly after releasing digital pressure. Although histological studies[12] confirm the vessels to be venular in origin, they are intimately associated with arterioles. Sclerotherapy of these vessels therefore requires considerable care to avoid cutaneous necrosis resulting from inadvertent intraarteriolar injection. Relapse following treatment is common.[13]

Cutis Marmorata Telangiectatica Congenita

Cutis marmorata telangiectatica congenita (CMTC) refers to a congenital pattern of prominent capillaries and venules that results in a bluish red mottling of the skin.[14] Physiological cutis marmorata is the cutaneous marbling effect seen in infants when they are exposed to cold. In contrast, the lesions of CMTC are more striking and independent of environmental temperature. Lesions may be generalized or localized; the lower limbs are most commonly affected (Fig. 1-4). The lesions are usually noted soon after birth and generally remain stable or fade significantly over several years. This is in contrast with nevus flammeus in which the vessels usually undergo progressive ectasia with lesions becoming progressively nodular and darker. More females than males have CMTC, and 50% of those affected have other congenital anomalies.[15] The most common associated

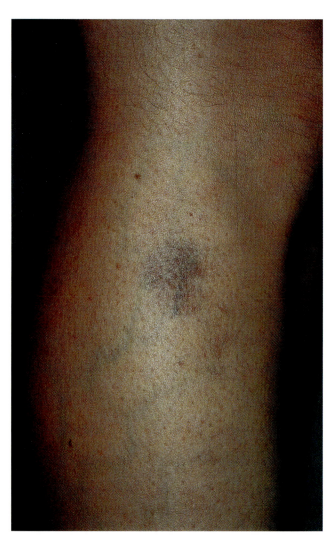

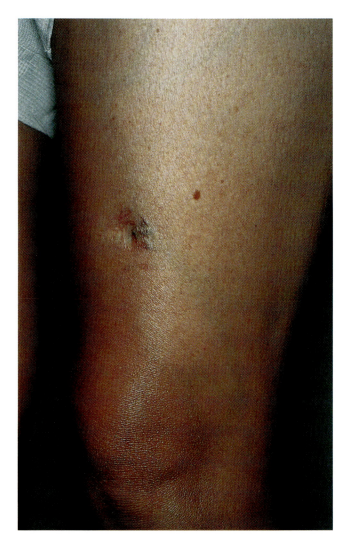

Fig. 1-5. A localized area of telangiectases that developed on the lateral aspect of the proximal calf several days after a contusion injury. This was the first manifestation of lower limb venous disease. At presentation 15 years later there were bilateral dilated reticular veins and telangiectases.

Fig. 1-6. Localized telangiectases developing adjacent to a scar on the distal anterior thigh. Close inspection reveals an associated dilated reticular vein draining towards the lateral aspect of the knee.

defects are hypoplasia or hyperplasia of an affected or unaffected limb, nevus flammeus, subcutaneous atrophy, and glaucoma. Most cases of CMTC occur sporadically and a multifactorial (autosomal dominant with low penetrance or teratogenic) etiology has been suggested.[15]

Localized Traumatic Telangiectasia

Soft tissue injuries can result in a susceptible individual suddenly developing a localized growth of telangiectases (Fig. 1-5). However, close inspection will usually reveal dilated subcutaneous reticular veins directly associated with the area of telangiectasia, as well as in noncontiguous areas and in the contralateral limb. Trauma may lead to the release of angiogenic mediators resulting in cutaneous neovascularization.[16]

These new vessels develop in a pattern similar to that of vessels already present in the area.[17] Apart from contusion injuries telangiectases may develop around scars as a result of an exaggerated angiogenic response to wound healing (Fig. 1-6).

Telangiectases Associated with Incompetence of the Lateral Venous System

The most common pattern of lower limb telangiectasia occurs on the lateral aspect of the thigh and is usually first noticed in the 20-to-40-year age group.[9] Females are usually affected and frequently have a family history of similar veins.[18] At the time of onset the telangiectases are unlikely to be associated with saphenous vein varicosities.[9] Typically they are noticed as a

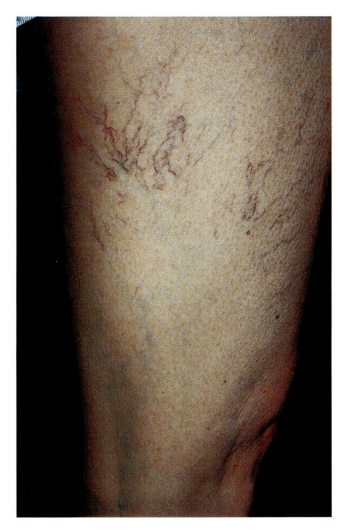

Fig. 1-7. Characteristic lateral thigh telangiectases forming the "cartwheel" pattern. In this patient the associated reticular veins drain to the popliteal fossa.

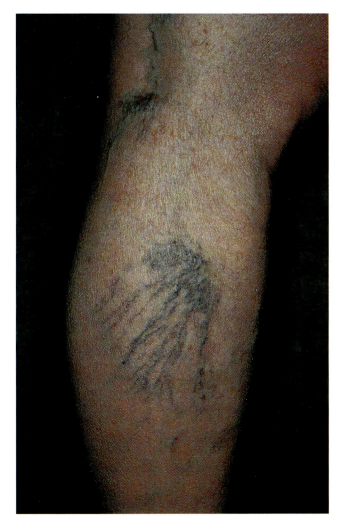

Fig. 1-8. Fan-shaped venulectases on the lateral thigh of a 57-year-old woman. These often appear as a reduced mirror image of the lateral thigh venulectases and arise from incompetence in the lateral venous system. These vessels are more prone to recurrent bleeding owing to the higher hydrostatic pressure in the calf veins.

radiating cartwheel appearance on the midlateral thigh (Fig. 1-7). In time they may extend around to the posterior thigh, and at this stage obvious associated reticular veins and small varices will be seen draining toward the popliteal fossa and lateral knee. Studies by Albanese and associates[19] and Weiss and Weiss[9] demonstrate incompetent perforating veins around the knee communicating with reticular veins associated with the posterolateral thigh telangiectases. These studies imply that perforating veins are instrumental in initiating incompetence in the lateral venous system. In contrast, Somjen and associates,[8] by analyzing the flows in the lateral venous system with high resolution duplex scanning, noted that direct perforating veins draining incompetent reticular veins, even if they did not display reflux, were relatively dilated owing to high volume flow from the incompetent reticular veins.

Incompetence in direct perforating veins therefore probably develops secondary to high volume reentry flow at a later stage of venous disease.

Coinciding with or some time after the initial appearance of lateral thigh telangiectases, telangiectases on the proximal to midlateral calf may be observed (Fig. 1-8). These result from the extension of reticular vein incompetence from the lateral knee region to the distal calf. Duplex imaging of lateral calf reticular veins and varices will reveal communications with dilated and at times incompetent soleal muscle perforating veins. Lateral leg telangiectases can also be associated with varicose anterior or posterior thigh accessory veins (Fig. 1-9). This process will be associated with extension of lateral thigh telangiectases to the anterior or posteromedial thigh.

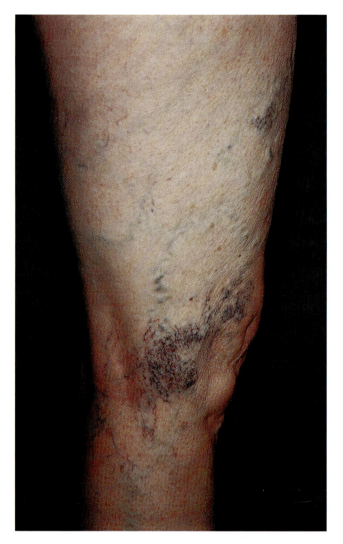

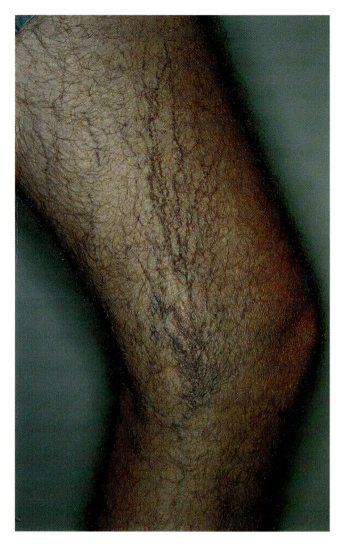

Fig. 1-9. Telangiectases on the lateral knee region associated with an incompetent anterior accessory branch of the long saphenous vein. Note that the distribution of the telangiectases is more distal than the usual location on the mid thigh. Duplex scanning in this patient revealed an incompetent long saphenous vein from the saphenofemoral junction to the distal calf.

Fig. 1-10. Medial thigh venulectases in a 52-year-old man with associated small varices draining to the proximal calf segment of the long saphenous vein. Duplex examination in this situation will frequently reveal segments of incompetence in the adjacent long saphenous vein, but with a competent saphenofemoral junction.

Telangiectases Associated with Incompetence in the Long Saphenous System

Telangiectases occurring on the medial aspect of the leg are frequently associated with incompetence in the long saphenous system.[20] Age of onset is generally later than with lateral venous system telangiectases and not infrequently occurs in men as well as women (Fig. 1-10). The first area usually affected will be the distal medial thigh where the telangiectases form a parallel linear pattern. Initially the associated incompetent reticular veins are difficult to observe in this area. As the telangiectases dilate with time, subcutaneous blue reticular veins will be observed both proximal and distal to the dermal lesions.

The appearance of telangiectases on the proximal medial calf should arouse suspicion of incompetence in the long saphenous vein and necessitate further evaluation with Doppler or duplex. An isolated area of telangiectasia on the posteromedial calf may indicate localized perforating vein incompetence, although this association is uncommon[11] (Fig. 1-11). More commonly reflux in the thigh segment of the long saphenous vein will also be contributing to dermal venous hypertension (Fig. 1-12).

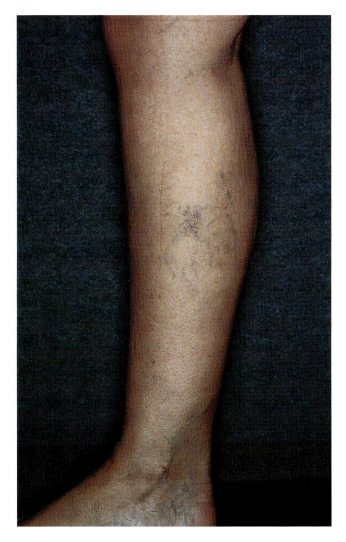

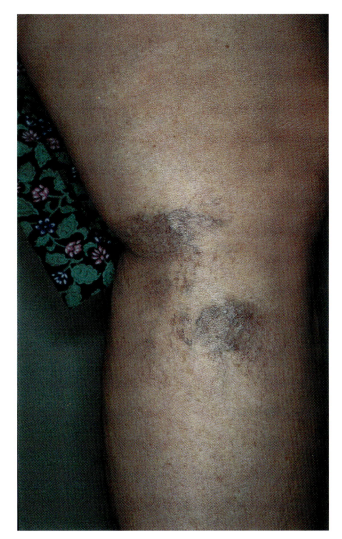

Fig. 1-11. An atypical area of telangiectasia on the midcalf. This was found by duplex examination to be receiving reflux from an incompetent distal calf posterior tibial perforating vein as well as an incompetent posterior arch vein that joined the long saphenous vein in the distal thigh. The main trunk of the long saphenous vein was competent from the saphenofemoral junction to the ankle. There was no deep venous insufficiency.

Fig. 1-12. Telangiectases on the proximal medial calf invariably denote a degree of incompetence in the long saphenous vein. In the absence of obvious truncal varices, the incompetence is generally segmental with a competent saphenofemoral junction.

Telangiectasia on the medial ankle or pedal area (corona phlebectasia) commonly has been associated with chronic venous hypertension or incompetence in the main trunk of the long saphenous vein (Fig. 1-13), although duplex examination occasionally reveals incompetence of saphenous vein tributaries with normal flows in the saphenous trunks and deep veins.

Telangiectases Associated with Incompetence of the Short Saphenous System

Occasionally, isolated areas of telangiectases will be the only evidence of short saphenous vein incompe-

tence (Fig. 1-14). If incompetence of the short saphenous vein is found by Doppler examination, duplex imaging will be required to determine whether the short saphenous vein terminates in the popliteal vein, deep in the posterior thigh muscles, or as a branch of the thigh segment of the long saphenous vein (Giacomini vein).

Telangiectases Developing After Surgery or Sclerotherapy for Varicose Veins

Previously unnoticed telangiectases can appear after sclerotherapy or surgical procedures for varicose veins and leg telangiectases. Fine telangiectases less

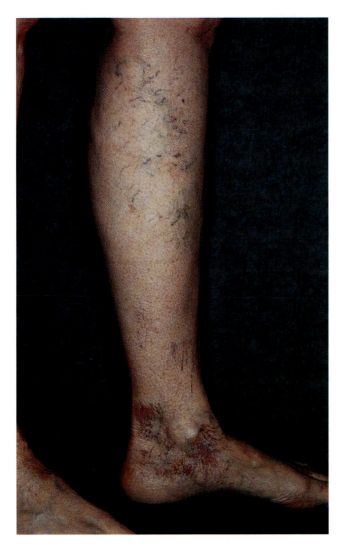

Fig. 1-13. Corona phlebectasia on the medial ankle in a 46-year-old woman. In this patient duplex examination revealed reflux in the calf segment of the long saphenous vein secondary to a communicating vein from an incompetent short saphenous vein and saphenopopliteal junction.

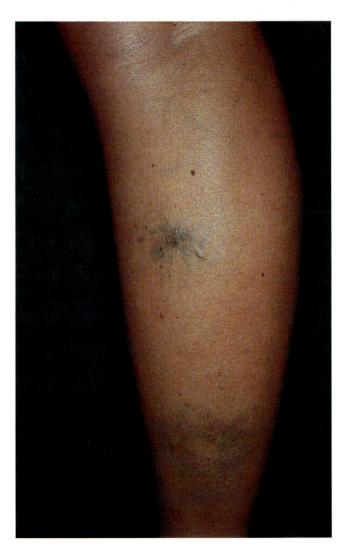

Fig. 1-14. The unusual distribution of telangiectases on the mid and distal calf aroused the suspicion of short saphenous vein incompetence in this 45-year-old woman. Duplex examination confirmed incompetence of the saphenopopliteal junction and short saphenous vein. There were no obvious varicose veins in this patient.

than 0.2 mm in diameter developing as a consequence of sclerotherapy are termed telangiectatic matting[21] (Fig. 1-15). Telangiectatic matting is likely related to persistence of dilatation and reflux in subcutaneous reticular and varicose veins. Common sites for developing telangiectatic matting are the medial and lateral thighs and lateral calf. These locations correspond to the sites where subcutaneous reticular vein dilatation first occurs.

Risk factors for telangiectatic matting are obesity, use of estrogen-containing hormones, and a family history of leg telangiectases.[22] Estrogen is a potent angiogenic hormone, so taking estrogen hormones during sclerotherapy should be avoided.

REFERENCES

1. Goldman MP and Bennett RG: Treatment of telangiectasia: A review, J Am Acad Dermatol 17:167-182, 1987.

2. Weiss RA and Weiss MA: Painful telangiectasias, their diagnosis and management. In Bergan JJ and Goldman MP, editors: Varicose veins and telangiectasias: Diagnosis and management, St Louis, 1993, Quality Medical Publishing.

3. Thibault PK: Treatment of telangiectasias. In Bergan JJ and Goldman MP, editors: Varicose veins and telangiectasias: Diagnosis and management, St Louis, 1993, Quality Medical Publishing.

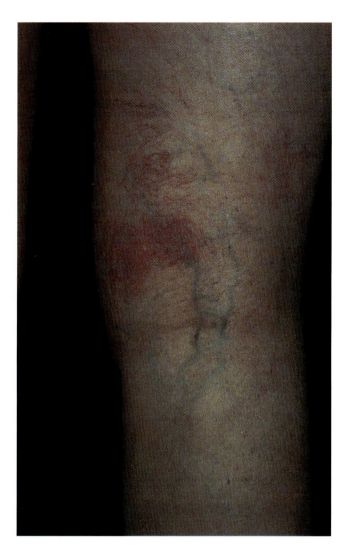

Fig. 1-15. Extensive telangiectatic matting developed on the posteromedial calf of this 47-year-old woman soon after sclerotherapy to residual postsurgical (long saphenous vein stripping) varicose veins. Note the persistence of small varicose and reticular veins in the popliteal fossa.

4. de Faria JL and Moraes IN: Histopathology of the telangiectasia associated with varicose veins, Dermatologica 127:321-324, 1963.

5. Wokalek H, Vanscheidt W, Martay K, and Leder O: Morphology and localisation of sunburst varicosities: An electron microscopic and morphometric study, J Dermatol Surg Oncol 15:149-154, 1989.

6. Tretbar LL: The origin of reflux in incompetent blue reticular/telangiectasia veins. In Davy A and Stemmer R, editors: Phlebologie '89, Paris, 1989, John Libbey Eurotext, Ltd.

7. Goldman MP: Commentary: Rational sclerotherapy techniques for leg telangiectasia, J Dermatol Surg Oncol 19:933, 1993.

8. Somjen GM, Ziegenbein R, Johnston AH, and Royal JP: Anatomical examination of leg telangiectases with duplex scanning, J Dermatol Surg Oncol 19:940-945, 1993.

9. Weiss RA and Weiss MA: Doppler ultrasound findings in reticular veins of the thigh subdermic lateral venous system and implications for sclerotherapy, J Dermatol Surg Oncol 19:947-951, 1993.

10. Sadick NS. Predisposing factors of varicose and telangiectatic leg veins, J Dermatol Surg Oncol 18:883-886, 1992.

11. Thibault P, Bray A, Wlodarczyk J, and Lewis W: Cosmetic leg veins: Evaluation using duplex venous imaging, J Dermatol Surg Oncol 16:612-618, 1990.

12. McGrae JD and Winkelmann RK: Generalized essential telangiectasia, JAMA 185:909-913, 1963.

13. Goldman MP: Pathophysiology of telangiectasias. In Goldman MP, editor: Sclerotherapy: Treatment of varicose and telangiectatic leg veins, St Louis, 1991, Mosby-Year Book.

14. Kurczynski TW: Hereditary cutis marmorata telangiectatica congenita, Pediatrics 70:52-53, 1982.

15. Picascia DD and Esterly NB: Cutis marmorata telangiectatica congenita: Report of 22 cases, J Am Acad Dermatol 20:1098-1104, 1989.

16. Ryan TJ: Factors influencing the growth of vascular endothelium in the skin, Br J Derm 82, Supp 5:99-108, 1970.

17. Ryan TJ and Kurban AK: New vessel growth in the adult skin, Br J Derm 82, Supp 5:92-98, 1970.

18. Hirai M, Naiki K, and Nakayama R: Prevalence and risk factors of varicose veins in Japanese women, Angiology 41:228-232, 1990.

19. Albanese AR, Albanese AM, and Albanese EF: The lateral subdermic varicose vein system of the legs, Vasc Surg 3:81-89, 1969.

20. Böhler-Sommeregger K, Karnel F, Schuller-Petrovic S, and Santler R: Do telangiectases communicate with the deep venous system?, J Dermatol Surg Oncol 18:403-406, 1992.

21. Duffy DM: Small vessel sclerotherapy: An overview. In Callen JP et al., editors: Advances in dermatology, vol 3, Chicago, 1988, Year Book Medical Publishers, Inc.

22. Davis LT and Duffy DM: Determination of incidence and risk factors for postsclerotherapy telangiectatic matting of the lower extremity: A retrospective analysis, J Dermatol Surg Oncol 16:327-330, 1990.

2

LABORATORY EVALUATION OF THE PATIENT WITH CHRONIC VENOUS INSUFFICIENCY

Hugo Partsch

Chronic venous insufficiency (CVI) is a pathophysiological term meaning failure to reduce pressure in peripheral veins of the leg during walking. Causes of this malfunction include venous reflux due to valvular incompetence, (partial) obstruction of deep veins, or a defect of the muscle pump. By Widmer's definition, the clinical consequences can be seen on the distal lower leg, mainly in the inner ankle region.[1] These include Stage I (edema, dilated venules, "corona phlebectatica," ankle flare); Stage II (lipodermatosclerosis, hyperpigmentation, stasis dermatitis); and Stage II (venous ulcer or ulcer and scar). These clinical signs can be associated with different kinds of varicose veins and subjective symptoms, but also can occur without any of these.

■ CLINICAL EVALUATION

Various clinical entities can be differentiated into Widmer's classifications just by inspection without any supplementary investigations. However, if we wish more detailed information concerning underlying pathophysiology and adequate swelling, some objective methods play an essential role.

■ CONTINUOUS-WAVE DOPPLER

Doppler ultrasound is the most important method in clinical practice today for assessing the patency of the large arteries of an extremity. It is also a very simple and reliable method for detecting venous reflux and helps assess venous obstruction. Bidirectional instruments that detect flow-direction are recommended for venous investigation.

For diagnosing venous reflux,[2] the patient is preferably in an upright position (sitting or standing). As a routine, the following sites are investigated: (1) Superficial veins including the greater saphenous vein (GSV) at the junction and along its course, the lesser saphenous vein (LSV) in the popliteal fossa and distally, and perforating veins; and (2) deep veins including the femoral vein in the groin, the popliteal vein, the posterior tibial vein behind the inner malleolus, and the anterior tibial vein accompanying the anterior tibial artery.

When the patient is in an upright position, spontaneous flow cannot be detected by an 8 to 10 MHz Doppler probe. Augmented flow in the proximal venous segments can be elicited by distal manual compression of the leg which will be followed by reflux through incompetent valves after release of the compression. Venous reflux can also be produced by deep inspiration or by a Valsalva's maneuver. This indicates incompetent valves proximal to the auscultation site (Fig. 2-1). In contrast to duplex scanning, it may be difficult to identify clearly the blood vessel from which the Doppler sound is detected. This can be especially true for the junctions of the long and short saphenous veins. Tapping distal parts of these veins which produce augmented flow waves may be helpful.

To identify the popliteal or the posterior tibial vein, we look for the arterial signal. The accompanying vein can be assessed by provoking an augmented venous flow by distal manual compression. To detect incompetent perforators, reflux via incompetent superficial veins has to be blocked by a tourniquet (Figs. 2-2 and 2-3). The incidence of false-positive tests is too high to rely on this technique as a guide for surgery.

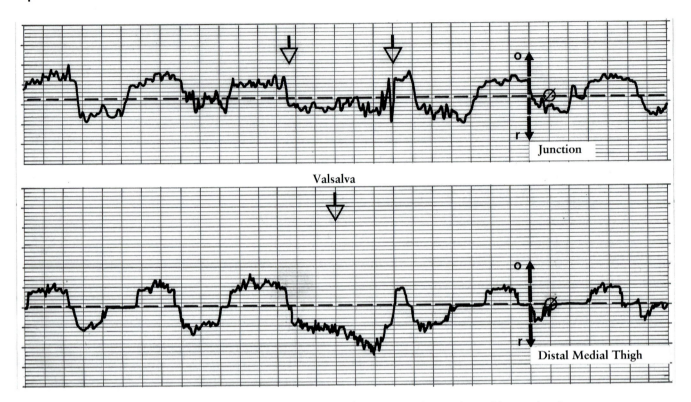

Fig. 2-1. Doppler ultrasonography with two-directional instruments in a patient with complete incompetence of the long saphenous vein. One probe is placed over the junction (upper curve) and the other over the distal medial thigh. The dashed horizontal line represents zero flow. The "o" indicates orthograde flow toward the heart and "r" indicates retrograde flow. With deep breathing (left half of the figure) and also during a Valsalva's maneuver (center), retrograde flow due to valvular incompetence can be detected at both sites.

Proximal Venous Obstruction

Proximal flow hindrance can be detected mainly by observing the spontaneous venous flow modulated by the breathing action of the abdomen.[3] If local venous pressure is increased due to proximal venous obstruction, continuous flow is detected that is not influenced by the excursion of the abdominal wall during respiration. When compared with the contralateral, healthy side, this kind of flow pattern may give a reliable estimate of an obstruction of the external or common iliac vein (a Doppler probe over the femoral vein in the groin, Fig. 2-4). With this technique, experienced investigators can also diagnose occlusion in the common and superficial femoral vein when auscultating the popliteal vein. Detection of venous flow patterns in collateral veins may increase accuracy of the Doppler examination regarding the diagnosis of venous occlusions. This kind of investigation still has some value in screening for deep venous thrombosis (DVT). According to our experience in 241 patients with iliac vein

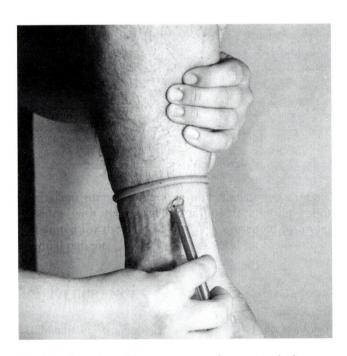

Fig. 2-2. Detection of incompetent perforators in the lower leg by Doppler ultrasound. A tourniquet is placed proximal to the auscultation site to impede superficial reflux. Over the incompetent perforator, reflux can be registered during compression of the calf or by tiptoeing.

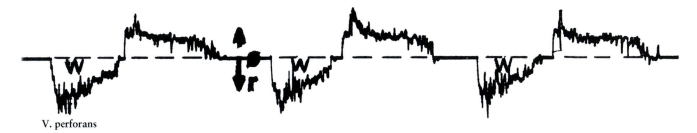

V. perforans

Fig. 2-3. Manual compression of the calf ("W") proximal to the tourniquet produces a retrograde flow in the incompetent perforator directed toward the Doppler probe. Release of the compression is followed by an orthograde flow (curve above the dashed zero line).

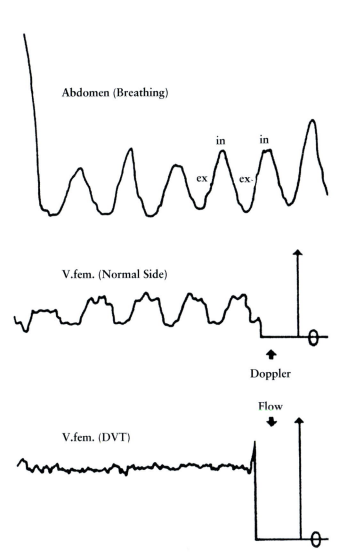

Abdomen (Breathing)

in   in

ex   ex

V.fem. (Normal Side)

Doppler

Flow

V.fem. (DVT)

0

Fig. 2-4. The upper curve represents respiratory movement of the abdomen. Simultaneous detection of venous flow of both femoral veins in a patient with unilateral iliac vein obstruction shows a homogeneous flow pattern without modulation by breathing on the pathologic side (lowest curve), inspiratory stop, and flow during expiration on the healthy side (middle curve).

obstruction, the sensitivity of this technique was 93.3% with a specificity of 80.7%.

Arterial Occlusive Disease

The assessment of arterial occlusion is based mainly on measuring blood pressure in different levels of the limb. Systolic ankle pressure is measured by placing a cuff at the distal lower leg or ankle when the patient is in the supine position.[4,5] The cuff is inflated to a suprasystolic value and released slowly. The first sound that can be detected by the Doppler instrument over the posterior tibial artery or the dorsalis pedis artery indicates the systolic ankle pressure. The ankle and brachial index ("Doppler index") is the quotient between systolic ankle pressure divided by the systolic brachial pressure. In normal situations, this index should be greater than one. Arterial stenoses with a reduction of the vessel diameter less than 70% do not cause a distal pressure reduction. After a stress test such as 20 tiptoe movements, there is a reduction in the systolic ankle pressure which persists for more than one minute in cases of significant arterial occlusion.

More detailed information regarding multilevel measurement, registration, and evaluation of arterial pulse curves, including frequency analysis can be gained from various textbooks.[6]

Bidirectional instruments with a frequency between 7 and 10 MHz are preferred. The most important and frequently asked clinical questions that can be answered by the Doppler include the following:

1. Is the long/short saphenous vein, including its junction, competent or incompetent?

2. Is there reflux in the deep veins?

3. Is the venous outflow proximal to the groin impeded?

4. Are there arterial obstructions in the large arteries?

The continuous-wave Doppler examination is an essential step assessing for every patient who has signs and symptoms of advanced stages of venous insufficiency.

■ PHOTOPLETHYSMOGRAPHY (PPG)

Various systems of PPG are on the market and give valuable information about the quality of the venous pump.[5]

Examination techniques consist of a probe attached preferably to normal-appearing skin above the inner malleolus using a double-adhesive tape and avoiding pressure-producing external fixation. The patient sits on a chair in a room at 20 to 24 degrees centigrade with bare feet on a towel to avoid direct contact with the cold floor. Between 8 and 20 dorsiflexions (averaging one per second) are performed. Changes of the local blood volume in the skin caused by the ankle movement are registered on a recorder. In a normal subject, every movement of the ankle will produce a shift of blood that is expelled up the veins toward the heart. Competent valves will prevent reflux so that blood volume in the peripheral veins and venules of the leg decreases. After stopping the exercise, blood will fill up the veins again by arterial inflow. The time needed for the volume curve to reach its plateau is called filling time (normal valves > 20 seconds).

In a patient with incompetent valves, blood will oscillate in the veins during exercise so that there will be only minor decreases of blood volume in the peripheral veins and venules. The veins are filled again quickly after stopping ankle movements. This is by arterial inflow and especially by venous reflux so that refill time will be shorter.

Tourniquet occlusion, or even better digital compression of incompetent superficial veins or of incompetent perforators, can help predict the functional benefit of removing incompetent veins. Small tourniquets, or the fingers, are used to compress the "leakage points" (incompetent saphenous junctions or perforators, Fig. 2-5).

The most important information that can be obtained using PPG is whether CVI in an individual patient can be improved by surgery or sclerotherapy of superficial veins and perforators as opposed to deep venous abnormalities.

An algorithmic flowchart is shown in Fig. 2-6. It is possible by this simple pattern to select candidates for treatment of incompetent veins by surgery or sclerotherapy. This information can have considerable clinical importance in patients with recurrent venous ulcerations. Other indications for PPG include functional assessment of therapy, screening for DVT, and differential diagnosis of the swollen leg.

Limitations of PPG should always be considered. From changes of a very small dermal blood volume, conclusions are drawn regarding the hemodynamics of the whole limb. The method depends to a considerable degree on arterial flow and ambient temperature. Reproducibility is marginal when measuring at different sites. PPG cannot be used to make a diagnosis. Normal refill times do not exclude venous disease. Shortened refill time does not necessarily indicate venous insufficiency. These restrictions are also true for the new cali-

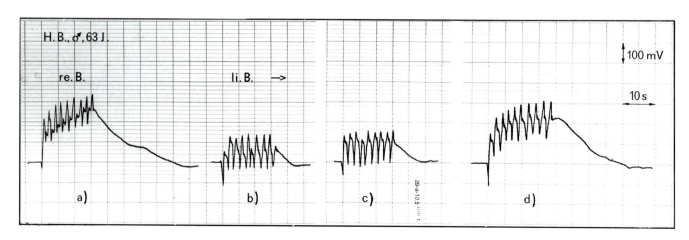

Fig. 2-5. Photoplethysmography with the probe above the inner malleolus. With 10 ankle dorsiflexions, there is an increase of light reflection due to normal venous emptying on the normal right leg (a), but not on the left leg with chronic venous insufficiency (b). With digital occlusion of the long saphenous vein in the proximal thigh, there is no improvement of venous pumping function (c). Normalization of the pumping curve by compression of Boyd's perforating vein (d).

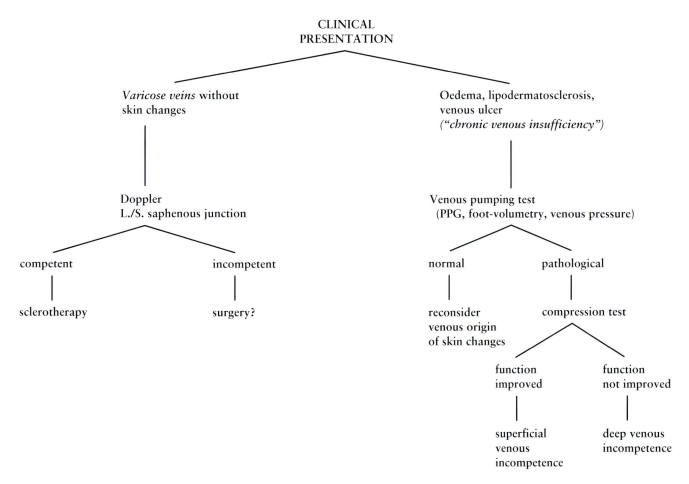

Fig. 2-6. This algorithm does not mean that Doppler and "pumping tests" are mutually exclusive in the diagnosis of varicose veins with and without skin changes. Our intention is to highlight the practical and deciding questions in a patient with venous disease.

brated systems[6] which are able to quantify refill time and relative expelled volume.

▮ Foot Volumetry, Strain-Gauge Plethysmography of the Foot

Other plethysmographic tests of the venous pump include foot volumetry and strain-gauge plethysmography of the foot.

Foot volumetry equipment is now difficult to acquire. In principle, it consists of a container filled with warm water (30 degrees).[8] The main advantages are the constant temperature and ability to measure expelled volume in milliliters using a simple calibration system. Since total foot volume is measured, expelled volume per 100 ml and the amount of refill volume per minute can be calculated (Fig. 2-7). Strain-gauge plethysmography of the foot can measure relative volume decrease (ml/100 ml) during exercise.[9]

The sample volume measured with these methods is much larger compared to PPG so these tests reveal more representative parameters of venous hemodynamics of an entire leg. In daily practice, PPG is often preferred because of its quick and easy application. The most important practical information gained with these two methods is the differentiation between superficial and deep venous insufficiency (Fig. 2-6).

▮ Venous Occlusion Plethysmography, Impedance Plethysmography

These methods are generally used for screening of DVT. The venous outflow of the elevated limb is blocked by a cuff at thigh level, and the volume increase of the calf is measured (so-called "venous capacitance") after several minutes (Fig. 2-8). The rate of volume decrease per time (ml 100 ml/min) after sudden

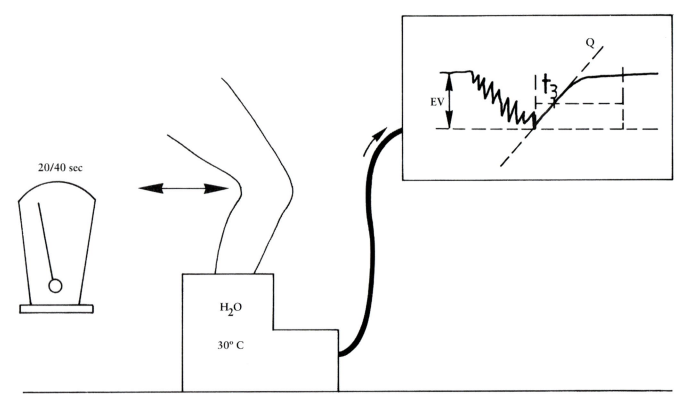

Fig. 2-7. Principle of foot volumetry. The feet are introduced into a container with warm water of 30 degrees centigrade. With 20 kneebends at 40 seconds, there is a decrease of foot volume due to the amount of blood pumped up toward the heart ("expelled volume" EV).

release of the cuff is a parameter for venous outflow resistance.[9,10] Both parameters, venous capacitance and venous drainage, decrease in acute proximal deep vein thrombosis (Fig. 2-9).

With impedance plethysmography, the resistance of a leg to an electric current is measured. This is indirectly proportional to its blood content. The equipment developed by Wheeler[11] can be transported to the patient's bedside. Venous capacitance and venous outflow are plotted on a special graph that contains a "discriminant line" separating normal from abnormal values.

For assessing a patient with signs of CVI, these methods can be of interest if the functions of recanalization and collateralization after DVT are to be quantified. Since venous capacitance and venous drainage have reached the normal range several months after acute DVT in most instances, both methods are *not* useful for the practical diagnosis of a postthrombotic syndrome.

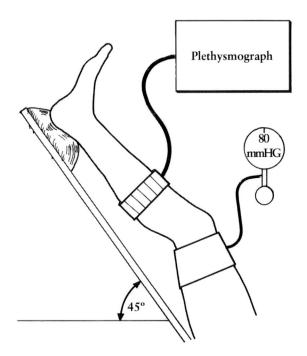

Fig. 2-8. Venous occlusion plethysmography is used mainly as a screening method for deep vein thrombosis. The leg is elevated and a mercury-filled strain gauge is placed around the calf. Volume changes of the calf are measured during and after venous occlusion on the distal lower thigh with a cuff.

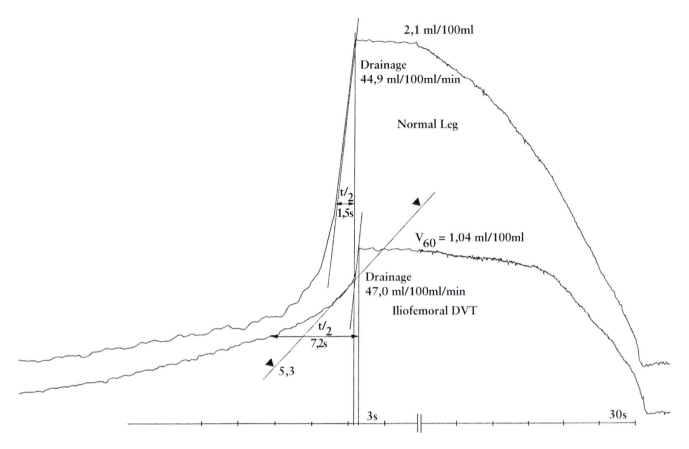

Fig. 2-9. Strain-gauge plethysmography in a patient with isolated iliac vein occlusion (no thrombi in the popliteal and femoral vein, lower curve). Curves are to be read from the right to the left. In comparison with the normal leg (upper curve), venous capacitance (V60) is diminished. The slowing of the venous-emptying rate after cuff deflation is flattened in the DVT leg (prolonged t/2). However, maximal venous outflow ("drainage") measured by the steepest tangent to the curve is even higher, pointing to an unimpeded outflow in the popliteal and femoral segment.

■ AIR PLETHYSMOGRAPHY (APG)

This method was introduced by Nicolaides' group and measures volume changes of the entire lower leg using an air-filled plastic bag wrapped around the calf.[12] Venous capacitance and venous outflow can be measured using the venous occlusion technique as well as the parameters characterizing the venous pump function.

Meaningful parameters that can be measured only by APG are the venous volume and venous filling index. Venous volume is defined as the difference between the plethysmographic reading with elevated legs (venous volume zero) and the volume during standing. The venous filling index (VFI) is defined as the ratio of 90% of the venous volume divided by the time taken to achieve 90% of filling (ml/sec). This parameter gives quantitative information on venous reflux. With competent valves, the volume increase of the lower leg is less than 2 ml/sec and reflects the filling of the veins by arterial inflow. Incompetent valves will cause reflux leading to a rapid volume increase. A VFI greater than 7 ml/sec is associated with a high incidence of skin changes typical for DVI. Applying a narrow tourniquet that occludes the superficial veins will reduce VFI to less than 5 ml/sec. in the limbs with primary varicose veins and competent popliteal veins. However, this test is subject to the errors inherent in all tourniquet tests.

Very comprehensive quantitative data concerning venous outflow obstruction, valvular function, and venous pumping efficacy can be obtained by APG. When reflux is excluded in the long saphenous vein by placing a tourniquet at thigh level, a complex functional evaluation of the individual patient is possible. Practical indications noted earlier for the PPG are applicable to APG. The abolition of venous reflux by compression can be measured in quantitative terms (Fig. 2-10). However, when comparing results of the

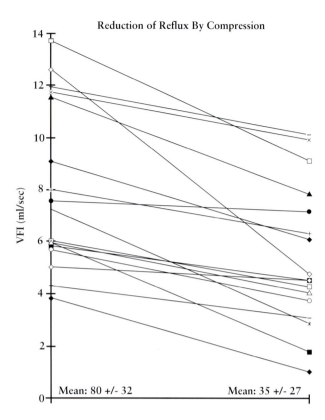

Fig. 2-10. Seventeen patients with venous leg ulcers were investigated by APG with and without calf compression stockings. As can be seen, there is a decrease of the venous filling index (VFI) by external compression in every case (average from 8.0 ± 3.2 ml/sec to 5.35 ± 2.7 ml/sec - Wilcoxon test: p < 0.01). This is explained by a reduction of venous reflux in both superficial and deep veins.

different methods of evaluation of venous pump function, one must remember that each method measures volume changes in different parts of the leg.

■ Venous Pressure Measurement

Measuring the pressure in a dorsal foot vein by using a needle or catheter connected to an electromagnetic transducer was considered the told standard for assessing venous pump function. Under normal conditions, peripheral venous pressure falls during walking—from about 80 to 100 mmHg in the standing position to approximately 10 to 30 mmHg.[13] Venous dysfunction is characterized by a lesser amount of pressure decrease. This causes increased pressure value during walking (> 50 mmHg) as compared with a healthy subject. This "ambulatory venous hypertension" is the functional substrate of chronic venous insufficiency since it triggers clinical consequences of edema, pigmentation, lipodermatosclcrosis, and ulcration.

In daily practice, direct peripheral pressure measurement has been replaced by the various noninvasive methods mentioned above. Its main indication is assessment of venous pump function with and without occlusion of superficial reflux. Fig. 2-11 shows functional improvement of the venous pump mechanism by a medical compression stocking. Elevated ambulatory venous pressure is associated with a high incidence of ulceration.[12] To quantify the severity of venous outflow obstruction, Raju recommends measuring the arm and foot differential.[14]

■ B-Mode Imaging, Duplex Scanning, Color-Flow Imaging

Ultrasonic B-scanning combined with pulsed Doppler flow investigation allows both for anatomical and functional assessment of the superficial and deep leg veins. The experienced investigator will be able to determine whether chronic venous insufficiency is caused by obstruction, reflux, or both.

With the patient preferably in the standing or semi-erect position, diameter of the veins, flow velocity, and flow rate can be measured. Different methods to quantify reflux in individual veins have been advocated: valve close time, venous reflux index, and velocity at peak reflux.[12,15] Retrograde flow can be elicited by a Valsalva's maneuver or decompression of a distal limb segment by tourniquet as described in detail in the chapter by van Bemmelen.

Deep vein visualization while the patient is horizontal may reveal occluded segments, partially recanalized lumens, and irregular vein walls. The examination can also help localize the site where the short saphenous vein joins the popliteal vein (Fig. 2-12) and detect incompetent perforators. Color duplex scanning makes the orientation much easier so that the time for investigating a limb can be shorter (Fig. 2-13). Duplex scanning also provides information about reflux in specific veins. The investigation is done with the patient upright. The sites to be studied are imaged with a 5 or 7.5 MHz probe. Manual calf compression or, preferably, a rapidly deflatable cuff is used. Localized and generalized reflux throughout the superficial or deep venous system can be identified.

Quantifying reflux is time consuming. Reflux time should not exceed 0.5 seconds. When peak reflux is greater than 15 ml/sec, regardless of whether such reflux is in the superficial or deep veins, the incidence of skin changes on the lower leg is high.[16]

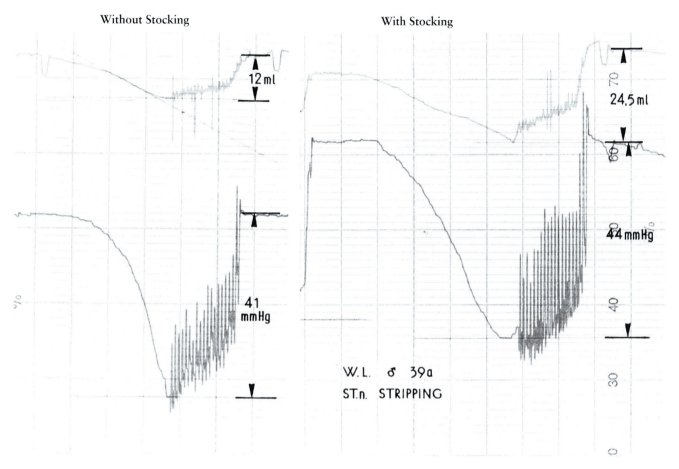

Without Stocking

With Stocking

12 ml

24,5 ml

41 mmHg

44 mmHg

W.L. ♂ 39a
ST.n. STRIPPING

Fig. 2-11. Simultaneous measurement of foot volumetry (upper curves) and peripheral venous pressure (lower curves) in a patient with chronic venous insufficiency. The curves should be read from the right to the left side. Without compression (left), expelled volume is diminished (12 ml; normal is around 18 ml), and also pressure fall is decreased (41 mmHg; normal is **greater than** 50 mmHg). A compression stocking doubles expelled volume, but leads only to a very moderate improvement of the pressure curve. (There is no linear relationship between volume and pressure).

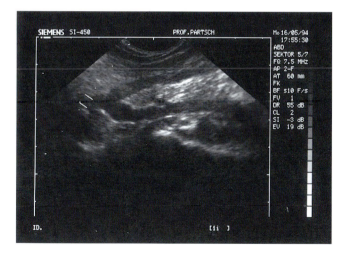

Fig. 2-12. B-scan of the short saphenous junction into the popliteal vein.

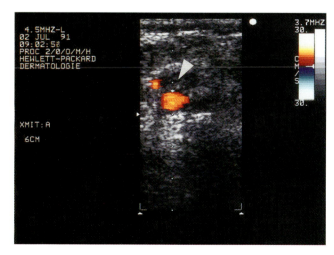

Fig. 2-13. Real-time color-flow imaging of the popliteal fossa. The red color indicates distal flow in the popliteal artery. No flow is detected in the popliteal vein which cannot be compressed and shows an occluding thrombus (*arrow*).

■ REFERENCES

1. Widmer LK, editor: Peripheral venous disorders, Bern, Stuttgart, Vienna, 1978, Hans Huber Publisher.

2. Folse R and Alexander RH: Directional flow detection for localizing venous vascular incompetency, Surgery 67:114, 1970.

3. Partch H. "A sounds" or "S sounds" for Doppler ultrasonic evaluation of pelvic vein thrombosis, VASA 5:16, 1976.

4. Yao JST, Hobbs JT, and Irvine WT: Ankle systolic measurements in arterial disease affecting the lower extremities, Br J Surg 56:676, 1969.

5. Bollinger A, Mahler F, and Gruntzig A: Peripheral haemodynamics in patients with coarctation, normotensive and hypertensive arteriosclerosis obliterans, Angiology 22:354, 1971.

6. Fronek A: Noninvasive diagnostics in vascular disease. New York, 1989, McGraw-Hill.

7. Flinn WR, Queral LA, Abramowitz HB, and Yao JST: Photoplethysmography in the assessment of chronic venous lower extremity. In Nicolaides AN and Yao JST, editors: Investigation of vascular disorders, New York, 1981, Churchill Livingstone.

8. Thulesius O, Norgren L, and Gjores JE: Foot volumetry: A new method for objective assessment of edema and venous function, VASA 2:325, 1973.

9. Barnes RW, Ross EA, and Strandness DE: Differentiation of primary from secondary varicose veins by Doppler ultrasound and strain-gauge plethysmography, Surg Gynecol Obstet 141:20, 1975.

10. Bygdeman S, Aschberg S, and Hindmarsh T: Venous plethysmography in the diagnosis of chronic venous insufficiency. Acta Chir Scand 137:423, 1971.

11. Wheeler HB and Penney BC: Impedance plethysmography: Theoretical and experimental basis. In Bernstein EF editor: Noninvasive diagnostic techniques in vascular disease. St Louis, 1978, Mosby.

12. Nicolaides AN and Sumner DS: Investigation of patients with deep vein thrombosis and chronic venous insufficiency, London, Los Angeles, Nicosia, 1991, Med-Orion.

13. Pollak AA and Wood EH: Venous pressure in the saphenous vein in the ankle of man during exercise and changes in posture, J App Physiol 1:649, 1949.

14. Raju S: New approaches to the diagnosis and treatment of venous obstruction, J Vasc Surg 4:42, 1986.

15. van Bemmelen PS, Bedford G, Beach K, and Strandness DE: Quantitative segmental evaluation of venous valvular reflux with duplex ultrasound scanning, J Vasc Surg 10:425, 1989.

16. Vasdekis SN, Clarke H, and Nicolaides AN. Quantification of venous reflux by means of duplex scanning, J Vasc Surg 10:670, 1989.

3

ULTRASOUND EXAMINATION OF THE PATIENT WITH VARICOSITIES

Paul S. van Bemmelen

Evaluating the patient with gross varicose veins can be relatively straightforward when the subcutis is thin. The greater and sometimes even the lesser saphenous veins can be palpated easily under those circumstances, and a portable Doppler examination can be performed with the patient standing and using release of distal compression.[1,2]

When thickness of the subcutis prevents accurate localization of veins, or if other indications exist, a duplex examination can be performed in the vascular laboratory.

◼ INDICATIONS FOR DUPLEX EXAMINATION FOR GROSS VARICOSE VEINS

The indications for this examination are as follows:

1. Obese patient
2. Recurrent varicose veins
3. Reflux in popliteal fossa by portable Doppler
4. Status, post deep venous thrombosis
5. Excessive subjective complaints
6. Severe stasis with skin changes
7. Surgical treatment

◼ TECHNIQUE OF STANDING DUPLEX EXAMINATION

The patient stands on a low stool and holds on to a walker. The standing position is important to promote closure of venous valves.[3,4] With the patient supine, a high percentage of tests would be false negative.[5] The knee is slightly flexed and weight placed on the contralateral leg. A large (24 cm width) cuff is placed on the thigh and connected to an automatic cuff inflator. The duplex probe is placed over the saphenofemoral junction. After the cuff has been inflated to 80 mmHg for three seconds, reflux is measured during cuff deflation.[6] This maneuver is repeated with the sample volume in the common femoral vein and superficial femoral vein just distal to its termination.

A 12 cm width cuff is placed below the knee, and the probe is placed over the saphenopopliteal junction. After inflation of the cuff to 100 mmHg for 3 seconds, reflux is measured during deflation of the cuff. The color duplex is an accurate technique to localize the termination of the lesser saphenous vein.[7] The sample volume is placed in the greater saphenous vein at the knee level, and cuff inflation and deflation are repeated.

The 12 cm cuff is lowered to the ankle level (Fig. 3-1) and the greater saphenous vein is examined at the calf level. At this level the greater saphenous vein often consists of two parts, the saphenous itself which originates anterior to the medial malleolus and the posterior arch vein—the vein of Leonardo.

The lesser saphenous vein is tested again at the midcalf level. If reflux is found at this level, with an intact saphenopopliteal junction, a search can be made for the Giacomini vein. With a good color scanner the deep calf veins can be tested using the same technique.

Next, a small (7 cm width) metatarsal cuff is placed around the foot. After inflation to 120 mmHg, reflux can be found in the ankle portion of the greater saphenous vein. This is less common than incompetence of the proximal portions of the greater saphenous vein. Reflux in incompetent pretibial branches can be demonstrated using this technique.

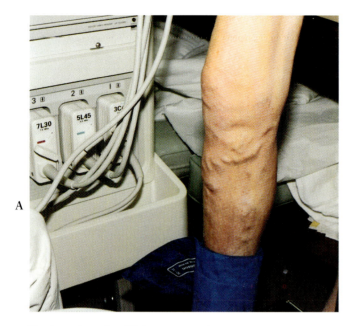

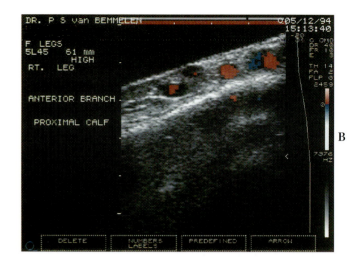

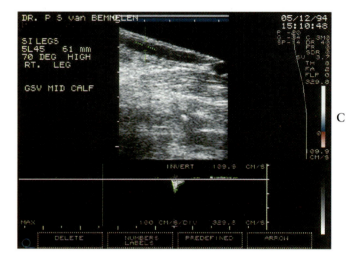

Fig. 3-1. A to C.   This greater saphenous vein was incompetent from the saphenofemoral junction to the below knee level. In spite of the clinical appearance of varicosities on the medial aspect of the calf, the greater saphenous vein in this area does not have pathological reflux with release of the cuff placed at the ankle. Antegrade flow toward the head is depicted below the base line. This patient could be a candidate for a limited stripping procedure of the greater saphenous vein from the groin to the knee.

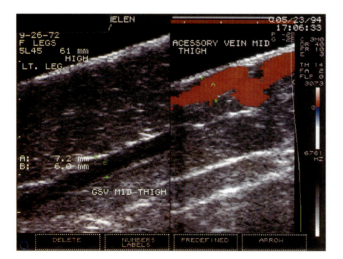

Fig. 3-2. This patient had large tortuous varicose veins on the medial aspect of the thigh. The saphenofemoral junction was incompetent. Surprisingly, the greater saphenous vein at the midthigh level is normal (left side of the split picture). The tortuous vein with reflux depicted in red is located more superficially (right half of the figure). This patient could be a candidate for high ligation and preservation of the intact greater saphenous vein.

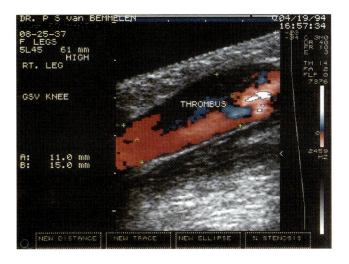

Fig. 3-3. This male patient suffered from several episodes of superficial phlebitis. The duplex examination confirmed greater saphenous incompetence and demonstrated residual thrombus in these side branches. At surgery these bulky veins could not be extracted with phlebectomy hooks, but required 2 cm long incisions for their removal.

REFERENCES

1. Nicolaides AN, Fernandes e Fernades J, and Zimmerman H: Doppler ultrasound in the investigation of venous insufficiency. In Nicolaides AN and Yao JST, editors: Investigation of vascular disorders, Chapter 28, New York, 1981, Churchill Livingstone.

2. Mitchell DC and Darke SG: The assessment of primary varicose veins by doppler ultrasound—the role of sapheno-popliteal incompetence and the short saphenous systems in calf varicosities, Eur J Vasc Surg 1:113-115, 1987.

3. van Bemmelen PS, Bedford G, Beach K, Isaac CA, and Strandness DE: Evaluation of tests used to document venous valve incompetence, J Vasc Technology 14:87-90,1990.

4. van Bemmelen PS, Beach K, Bedford G, and Strandness DE: The mechanism of venous valve closure, Arch Surg 125:617-619, 1990.

5. Foldes MS, Blackburn MC, Hogan J, Klemp K, Rutherford K, Thorpe L, and Auer AI: Standing versus supine positioning in venous reflux evaluation, J Vasc Technology 15:321 324, 1991.

6. van Bemmelen PS, Bedford G, Beach K, and Strandness DE: Quantitative segmental evaluation of venous valvular reflux with duplex ultrasound scanning, J Vasc Surg 10:425-431, 1989.

7. Vasdekis SN, Clarke GH, Hobbs JT, and Nicolaides AN: Evaluation of non-invasive and invasive methods in the assessment of short saphenous vein termination, Br J Surg 76:929-932, 1989.

Part II

Treatment of the Patient with Telangiectasias

4

DUPLEX ANATOMY OF TELANGIECTASIAS AS A GUIDE TO TREATMENT

George M. Somjen

As phlebology has been emerging in the nineties, there is a new emphasis on the "smaller end of the scale." The treatment of cosmetically disfiguring, often symptomatic telangiectasias and smaller varicose veins is gaining more acceptance.

The etiology of varicose veins can be multifactorial, but there is only one final common manifestation: the dilated venous conduit, with incompetent valves. The smallest valve containing venules, in which incompetence may occur, is situated in the lower dermis.

Telangiectasias, dilated intradermal veins, can develop as a result of long standing venous insufficiency. These patients may have the full range of venous pathology from large varicose veins to telangiectasias with extensive venous reflux in the superficial or deep venous systems.

Patients with minimal symptoms and primarily unsightly telangiectasias fall into a different category. One important etiological factor behind these "primary" telangiectasias is still high venous pressure due to valvular incompetence; however, the extent and distribution of reflux is limited. In cases of "primary" telangiectasia, without large "saphenous" varicose veins, reflux at the saphenofemoral or saphenopopliteal junction is less likely, but possible.[1] In most of these cases reticular vein reflux and perforating vein incompetence are associated with the telangiectatic blemishes.[2,3,4,5]

Accurate description of the anatomy of venous drainage from telangiectasias and evaluation of the extent of valvular incompetence are important factors when planning sclerotherapy.

Duplex ultrasonography is a unique diagnostic method that allows simultaneous morphological and functional examinations of blood vessels in the context of the surrounding tissues. Blood flow characteristics can be tested repeatedly, allowing the blood flow in the

same vessel to be observed under different conditions (change of position, augmentation, and so forth) and eventually functional anatomical information can be derived. With high definition imaging, anatomical structures close to the microscopic dimension can be interrogated, including the vascular system to the level of subdermal veins of less than 1 mm in diameter.

Most of the findings presented here were derived from our study, when duplex ultrasound examination of the subcutaneous venous anatomy was undertaken on legs with "primary" thigh telangiectasias.[3]

Our aim was to construct the functional map of the subcutaneous venous system and investigate the extent of subdermal venous incompetence associated with telangiectasias.

VENOUS ANATOMY OF THE SUBCUTANEOUS BLOOD VESSELS REVEALED BY THE DUPLEX ULTRASOUND

For accurate and uniform presentation of our findings the classification of subcutaneous veins are based on the "Revised Vessel Classification" suggested by Weiss and Weiss.[6] The vessels are categorized according to their size and appearance in increasing order: Type I, telangiectasias (blue to red); Type II, venulectasias; Type III, reticular veins; Types IV and V, nonsaphenous and saphenous varicose veins.

The Superficial Fascia and its Relation to the Subcutaneous Veins

The strong deep fascia envelops the calf and thigh muscles. The double layer of the superficial fascia in the subcutaneous layer is the distal continuation of the Camper's and Scarpa's fascias on the thigh. It covers and insheathes the long saphenous vein, anchoring it down to the deep fascia (Fig. 4-1).[7] The superficial facial appears as a strong reflective layer on the ultrasound. Normally it is seen as a continuous circumferential sheath on the thigh. Apart from the long saphenous vein and the proximal segments of the lateral and medial accessory saphenous veins, only the perforating veins can be located beneath the superficial fascia on the thigh. Tributaries of the long saphenous vein and other smaller subcutaneous veins (including reticular veins) are situated superficial to it. Varicose veins almost always occur above the superficial fascia (Figs. 4-1 and 4-2).[8] Its integrity on the thigh is well maintained even in patients with advanced varicose veins. (Below the knee, however, disintegration of the fascial structure may be seen with large varicose veins.) The lack of strong fascial support above the superficial fascia in the subcutaneous layer may be an important contributing factor in causing varicose veins.

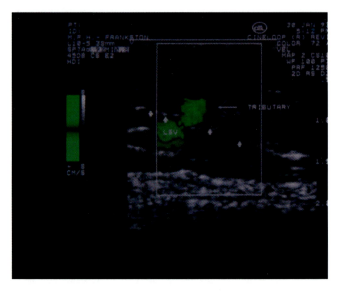

Fig. 4-1. Cross sectional view of the long saphenous vein in the thigh deep to the superficial fascia (superficial fascia is marked with arrows). A varicose tributary of the long saphenous vein is passing through the superficial fascia. The vein is narrowed at the fascia level. Varicose dilatation occurs only in the more superficial course of the tributary.

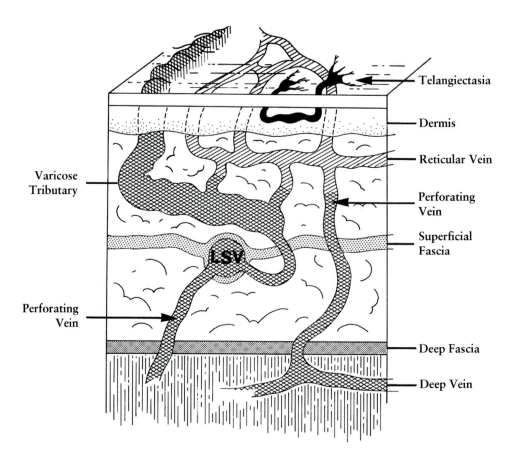

Fig. 4-2. Schematic diagram of the subcutaneous venous anatomy. The arrangement of the subcutaneous venous network is depicted in relation to the deep and superficial fascias. A network of communicating veins is displayed between veins of different types. Perforating veins arising from the long saphenous veins or from reticular veins, communicating with the deep veins beneath the deep fascia are also indicated.

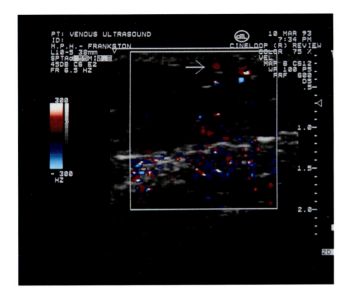

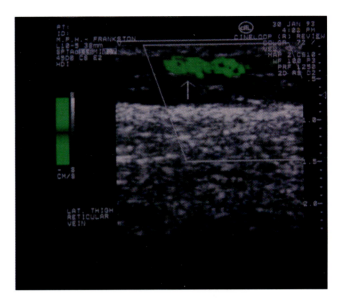

Fig. 4-3. A, Cross sectional view of subdermal venulectasia. Blood flow is indicated by blue color on compression augmentation. **B,** Reverse flow in venulectasia on compression release indicated by the red color. (Note: the numerous blue and red spots in the ultrasonic image are tissue movement artifacts.)

Fig. 4-4. Longitudinal view of reticular vein above the superficial fascia.

TELANGIECTASIAS (0.1-1 MM) AND VENULECTASIAS (1-2 MM)

Our study has indicated that in the presence of extensive thigh telangiectasias, the larger incompetent venules (Type II) can be seen in the dermis communicating with deeper reticular veins (Fig. 4-3). Telangiectasias and other venous structures less than 1 mm in diameter are rarely visualized by the ultrasound (10 MHz imaging transducer coupled with the 5 MHz pulsed Doppler probe).

RETICULAR VEINS (2-4 MM)

Reticular veins (Type III), frequently communicating with each other, usually run as a network parallel with the skin surface between the superficial fascia and the dermis-fat interface (Fig. 4-4). These veins also have numerous communications with larger veins (saphenous tributaries) above the superficial fascia and also with the deep veins through perforators (Fig. 4-2). Avalvular communicating venous segments exist between reticular veins and flow direction can change ("oscillate") in these veins under physiological circumstances.[9]

The three main drainage directions from the reticular veins can be followed on the thigh by the duplex scanner:

1. Toward the long and short saphenous veins.

2. Toward the deep veins of the thigh through perforating veins.

3. Toward the pelvic veins through the inferior gluteal vein as an alternative proximal drainage route of the lateral subdermic venous system (Fig. 4-5).[6,10]

The pattern of reticular vein arrangement is best examined on the lateral aspect of the thigh, where they are more numerous and not masked by the large saphenous tributaries. The longitudinal saphenous channels are dominant closer to the medial aspect of the thigh. Incompetent reticular veins, larger than 1.3 mm in diameter are easily recognizable with the help of color flow imaging (Fig. 4-6). Reticular vein incompetence is associated with thigh telangiectases in about 90% of the affected limbs.[3,4]

VARICOSE TRIBUTARIES (NONSAPHENOUS VARICOSE VEINS [3-8 MM] AND SAPHENOUS VARICOSE VEINS [>8 MM])

These individual varicose veins do not follow the interconnecting pattern of the smaller reticular veins, they are single tributaries running along the axis of the extremity predominantly above the superficial fascia. Often it is possible to trace their origin as they dive deeper beneath the superficial fascia, terminating in the saphenous "collecting" layer. Occasionally a sudden caliber change can be observed as they pass through the superficial fascia; varicose dilatation takes place in the more superficial course of the vein (Fig. 4-1).

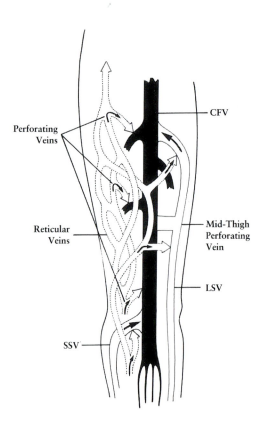

Fig. 4-5. Schematic representation of drainage pathways from the reticular veins of the thigh. The arrows indicate the drainage routes toward the long saphenous vein, short saphenous vein and the deep veins through perforators. The most proximal drainage of the lateral subdermic venous system (Albanese) is also indicated as an alternative path towards the pelvic veins.

■ PERFORATING VEINS

Perforating veins can be considered to be "direct" when they drain reticular veins and varicose tributaries straight to the deep system and "indirect" when they drain indirectly via the long or short saphenous systems.

Perforating veins, providing "direct" deep drainage from reticular veins, are small and numerous; they are situated along the lines of intermuscular septa. Their anatomical arrangement was extensively investigated by Taylor and associates.[9] Perforating veins play an important part in the venous drainage of the subcutaneous veins. The typical "stellate," segmental pattern of venous drainage through perforators is obscured by the alternative longitudinal arrangement of the long saphenous vein and tributaries.[9]

Perforating veins pass through the fascia layers (superficial and deep fascias) either in a short straight or a longer oblique course. They are frequently single (larger) perforating veins (Fig. 4-7), or they appear as small venae comitantes accompanying perforating arteries (Fig. 4-8). With high definition ultrasound, imaging the fine "direct" perforating veins is possible. Still, because of lack of sensitivity, especially color doppler sensitivity, many of the smaller (≤1 mm) veins remain undetectable. Direct perforating veins are visualized in 60% of limbs with extensive thigh telangiectasias. Bidirectional flow (reflux) is found in about half of the extremities with detected perforating veins (Somjen, unpublished data).

Reticular veins may also drain "indirectly" through the large perforators of the saphenous system (Hunterian, Dodd and Boyd perforators). These veins

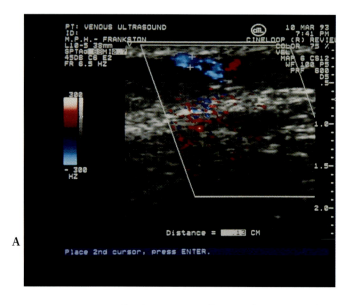

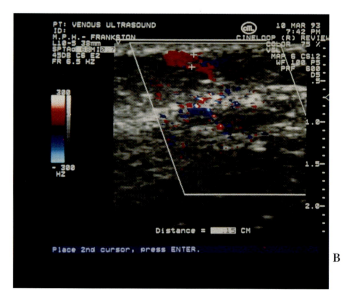

Fig. 4-6. A, Reticular vein draining venulectasia. Centripetal flow (blue) on augmentation.
B, Reverse blood flow on compression release, indicated by the change of color (red).

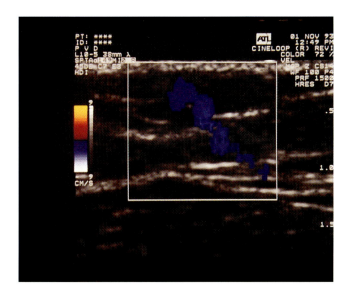

Fig. 4-7. Direct perforating vein arising from a reticular vein. After a tortuous and oblique path it pierces the deep fascia and joins the deep veins.

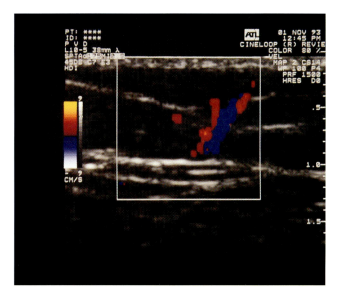

Fig. 4-8. Perforating vein arising from a reticular vein. This perforating vein runs a short, straight course and accompanies a subcutaneous artery (vena comitans).

are easily accessed for duplex ultrasound interrogation, and their role has already been widely studied.[11]

RETICULAR VEIN AND PERFORATING VEIN INCOMPETENCE ASSOCIATED WITH TELANGIECTASIAS: FUNCTIONAL CONSIDERATIONS

Reticular Vein Incompetence

Reticular vein incompetence is a usual feature associated with telangiectasia. With a large network of reticular veins, containing incompetent valves and valveless tributaries, blood flow "rearrangement" is likely when one changes from a supine to an upright position. Venous drainage in a supine patient may still be entirely centripetal (Fig. 4-5). While the patient is upright, when gravitational force comes into action, drainage to the distal direction is more likely (Fig. 4-9).

A distal direction of drainage in the reticular venous system is suggested in the standing position by the duplex scan examination. The distally flowing venous blood eventually reaches the first collecting venous conduit with competent valves "offering" centripetal blood flow. The likely pathways of reflux (distal drainage) from incompetent thigh reticular veins are listed on p. 34.

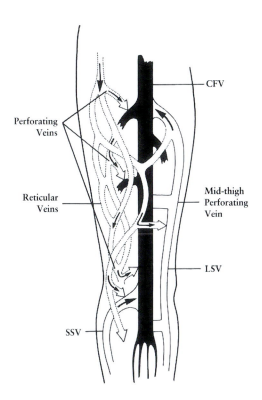

Fig. 4-9. Schematic representation of reverse drainage routes from incompetent reticular veins in standing position. The reverse flow in the incompetent reticular system eventually reaches "competent" veins directing the flow into centripetal direction. The perforating veins act as one way drainage channels.

a. From all aspects of the thigh, reticular veins may reach more distally situated segments of the long saphenous vein.

b. Perforating veins along the intermuscular septa collect the downward flowing blood and provide direct drainage toward the subfascial deep veins communicating with the superficial femoral vein, or profunda system. If any of the draining perforating veins develop valvular incompetence they can cease to serve solely as drainage routes. They will act as additional reflux sources further contributing to the reverse flow in the reticular system (Fig. 4-10).

c. When approaching the popliteal fossa, reticular veins drain into the proximal short saphenous vein via direct tributaries.

d. Further distally, below the knee, similar drainage patterns toward the deep veins and the distal saphenous veins occur.

Perforating Vein Incompetence

Most perforating veins reveal prolonged unidirectional flow toward the deep system after distal augmentation (in upright position), indicating the relatively large volume of blood pouring down from the incompetent reticular venous network (Fig. 4-9). Perforating veins displaying bidirectional flow (reflux) are found in about half of the extremities with detected perforating veins (Fig. 4-10). Reflux in the large, "saphenous" perforating veins of the thigh can further complicate the venous hemodynamics. The retrograde pressure effect on the reticular veins will be exerted "indirectly" via an incompetent long saphenous vein and its tributaries (Fig. 4-10). This manifestation can be seen in more advanced cases of varicose vein disease.

The exact role of perforating veins in developing varicose veins is still debated.[12] Their primary importance as reflux sources (subfascial escape points) has been stressed recently in relation to the lateral venous system of the thigh, based on continuous-wave Doppler studies.[4] Our recent work using the duplex ultrasound indicates that the "direct" perforating veins, which drain incompetent reticular veins, initially may serve as physiological, one-way entry channels, although coping with an increased blood flow during postural rearrangement of venous drainage. At a later stage they may become dilated and secondary (functional) incompetence occurs, as it was described in relation to large perforating veins of the leg.[13]

We can conclude from the functional anatomical studies that extensive telangiectasias mostly appear in areas where there is a dense, incompetent reticular venous network, and their pattern can relate somewhat to the anatomy of the direct perforating veins.

■ SUBCUTANEOUS ARTERIES

Subcutaneous arteries accompanied by perforating veins can often be visualized with the ultrasound (Fig. 4-8). In his recent work Salles-Cunha pointed out the likely influence of subcutaneous feeding arteries and veins, which were revealed by duplex ultrasound examination in the vicinity of telangiectasias.[14] More research is needed, however, regarding these arteries. At this time we cannot ascertain their significance in relation to telangiectasias.

■ CONCLUSION

Venous valvular incompetence is regarded as the major factor in developing varicose veins. Clinical symptoms and the appearance of varicose veins can vary depending on the anatomical distribution of reflux. With the wider application of duplex scan examination, a more elaborate localization of venous reflux can be provided which leads to better understanding of the pathophysiology of varicose veins.

High definition duplex ultrasound is a valuable research tool. It has shown us that telangiectasias appear in areas of significant reticular vein incompetence and has also indicated a relationship between direct perforating veins and telangiectases.

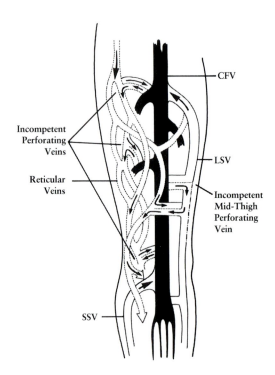

Fig. 4-10. Schematic illustration of reticular vein incompetence associated with perforating vein reflux. Arrows within perforating veins indicate bidirectional flow.

Clinical examination and continuous Doppler studies, however, should remain the mainstay of diagnostic workup before sclerotherapy of cosmetic leg veins and telangiectasias. Our findings further emphasize that injection sclerotherapy of telangiectasias should include the treatment of larger incompetent reticular veins to eliminate reflux and related high venous pressure affecting the dermal circulation.

■ REFERENCES

1. Thibault P, Bray A, Wlodarczyk J, and Lewis W: Cosmetic leg veins: evaluation using duplex venous imaging, J Dermatol Surg Oncol 16:612, 1990.

2. Goldman MP: Anatomy and histology of the venous system of the leg. In Goldman MP: Sclerotherapy: treatment of varicose and telangiectatic leg veins, St Louis, 1991, Mosby.

3. Somjen GM, Ziegenbein R, Johnston AH, and Royle JP: Anatomical examination of leg telangiectases with duplex scanning, J Dermatol Surg Oncol 19:940, 1993.

4. Weiss RA and Weiss MA: Doppler ultrasound findings in reticular veins of the thigh, J Dermatol Surg Oncol 18:62, 1992.

5. Tredbar LL: The origin of reflux in incompetent blue reticular/telangiectasia veins. In Davy A and Stemmer A, editors: Phlebologie '89, London, 1989, John Libbey Eurotext, Ltd.

6. Weiss AR and Weiss MA. Painful telangiectasias: diagnosis and treatment. In Bergan JJ and Goldman MP, editors: Varicose veins and telangiectasias, diagnosis and treatment, St Louis, 1993. Quality Medical Publishing, Inc.

7. Thomson H: The surgical anatomy of the superficial and perforating veins of the lower limb, Ann RCS of Eng 61:198, 1979.

8. Miller SS: Investigation and management of varicose veins, Ann Col Surg Eng 55:245, 1974.

9. Taylor GI, Caddy CM, Watterson PA, and Crock JG: The venous territories (venosomes) of the human body: Experimental study and clinical implications, Plast Reconstr Surg 86:185, 1990.

10. Albanese AR, Albanese Am, and Albanese EF: The lateral subdermic venous system of the legs, Vasc Surg 3:81, 1969.

11. Hanrahan LM, Araki CT, Fisher JB et al.: Evaluation of the perforating veins of the lower extremity using high resolution duplex imaging, J Cardiovasc Surg 32:87, 1991.

12. Sarin S, Scurr JH, and Coleridge Smith PD: Medial calf perforators in venous disease: The significance of outward flow, J Vasc Surg 16:40, 1992.

13. Bjordal RI: Circulation patterns in incompetent perforating veins of the calf in venous dysfunction. In May R, Partsch J, and Staubesand J, editors: Perforating veins. Munchen-Wien-Baltimore, 1981, Urban & Schwarzenberg.

14. Salles-Cunha SX. Telangiectasias: classification of feeder vessels using color flow duplex scanning. XXI World Congress, The International Society for Cardiovascular Surgery, Lisbon, Portugal, Sep 12-15, 1993 Abstract Volume pp 17-18.

5

SCLEROTHERAPEUTIC AGENTS AVAILABLE IN THE UNITED STATES AND ELSEWHERE

Margaret A. Weiss and Robert A. Weiss

INTRODUCTION TO SCLEROSING SOLUTIONS

One of the most often asked questions about performing sclerotherapy is which sclerosing solution to use in a particular situation. The typical answer is to use the solution with which a physician is most familiar. We have compared several solutions side by side in similar size vessels with similar sources of reflux. Some differences have emerged between categories of solutions, concentrations of solutions, and the sites at which these agents are injected.

The initial clue to proper choice of sclerosing solution is understanding the subtle differences in action mechanism. Some agents are potent initiators of damage to endothelial and muscular layers, whereas others produce very little more than endothelial cell disruption. Commonly used sclerosants have been classified into groups based on chemical structure or effect: hyperosmotic, detergent, and corrosive agents (chemical toxins—salts, alcohols, and acid or alkaline solutions) (Table 5-1). Sclerotherapy began, and was almost doomed to extinction, with caustic heavy metal salts such as ferric chloride. These irreversible bind to all proteins, causing extensive uncontrollable and indiscriminate tissue destruction as they corrode a vessel wall and penetrate surrounding tissues. Use of these agents has therefore been limited.

Hyperosmotic Solutions

Hyperosmotic solutions not only cause dehydration, destruction, and disintegration of the endothelium, but can also disrupt other layers of the vessel wall. The destruction of the endothelial layer is relatively slow (minutes) when compared to detergent solutions (seconds).[1] Of course, there is a direct correlation between osmotic concentration and depth of vein wall disruption (Table 5-2). Hyperosmotic solutions affect all cells in the path of the osmotic gradient. Nerve endings in the vessel adventitia or the underlying muscle may be stimulated, causing a burning pain or cramping sensation that lasts from seconds to minutes; the duration is rarely longer than five minutes.[2] Because an osmotic gradient weakens quickly by diffusion, this class of sclerosing solutions is effective primarily on smaller, more superficial vessels. Osmotic solutions are therefore considered milder solutions less capable of initiating a cascade of inflammation. This becomes important when examining side effects such as hyperpigmentation, thought to be related to inflammation leading to increased deposition of red blood cells into perivascular tissue (Fig. 5-1). Relative incidence of side effects is discussed later.

In situations in which the osmotic gradient may not be rapidly diluted, such as very close to the skin surface, damage of tissue adjacent to injection sites can easily occur. *Large ulcers can be produced by inadvertent dermal injection of hypertonic saline unless rapid dilution is undertaken.* Immediate intense pain upon extravasation accompanied by persistent white blanching warns against further injection at the site and is an indication for dilution. In our practice, this is performed with injection of a 10-fold volume of sterile water.

Hypertonic saline (Fig. 5-2). Although approved by the FDA only for use as an abortifacient, one of the most commonly employed hyperosmotic solutions is hypertonic saline (HS) at a concentration of 23.4%. The advantage of HS is its theoretical total lack of allergenicity when unadulterated. HS has been commonly used in various concentrations from 10-30%, with the addition of heparin, procaine, or lidocaine. A patented solution, Heparsal, containing 20% hypertonic saline,

Table 5-1   Important Characteristics of Sclerosing Solutions

Sclerosing Solution (Brand names)	Class	Allergenicity	Risks	FDA Approval	Dose Limitation Increased volume per session associated with increased risks of allergenicity
Hypertonic saline (HS)	Hyperosmotic	None	• Necrosis of skin • Pain and cramping	Yes, as abortifacient	6–10 ml (estimate based on authors' experience)
Hypertonic saline and dextrose (HSD) (**Sclerodex**)	Hyperosmotic	Low (due only to added phenethyl alcohol)	• Pain (much less than HS)	No (sold in Canada)	10 ml of undiluted solution
Sodium tetradecyl sulfate (STS) (**Sotradecol, S.T.D. Injection, Thromboject**)	Detergent	Rare anaphylaxis	• Pigmentation • Necrosis of skin (higher concentrations) • Pain with perivascular injection	Yes	10 ml of 3%
Polidocanol (POL) (**Aethoxysklerol, Aetoxisclerol, Sclerovein**)	Detergent	Rare anaphylaxis	• Lowest risks of necrosis • Lowest risks of pain • Pigmentation at higher concentrations	No	10 ml of 3%
Sodium morrhuate (SM) (**Scleromate**)	Detergent	Anaphylaxis, highest risk	• Pigmentation • Necrosis of skin • Pain	Yes	10 ml
Ethanolamine oleate (EO) (**Ethamolin**)	Detergent	Urticaria Anaphylaxis	• Pigmentation • Necrosis of skin • Pain • Viscous, difficult to inject	Yes (used primarily for esophageal varices)	10 ml
Polyiodide iodine (PII) (**Varigloban, Variglobin**)	Corrosive	Anaphylaxis Iodine hypersensitivity reactions	• Pain on injection • Necrosis of skin • Dark-brown color makes intravascular placement more difficult to confirm	No	5 ml of 3%
72% glycerin with 8% chromium potassium alum (CGLY)(**Chromex, Scleremo**)	Corrosive	Extremely rare anaphylaxis	• Ineffective sclerosis (weak agent) • Very low risks of necrosis • Lowest risk of pigmentation	No	5 ml (estimate)

100 units/cc of heparin, and 1% procaine was thought to reduce pain and prevent thrombus formation in deep vessels, but a recent study of 800 patients demonstrated that adding heparin to HS provided no benefit.[3] Though claims of pain reduction with procaine or lidocaine are exaggerated, HS is used either unadulterated or diluted to 11.7% with sterile water for smaller telangiectasias.[4] A high success rate with 23.4% HS in treating telangiectasias in nearly 300 patients with few complications has been previously reported.[2] Intense burning pain or muscle cramping immediately following injection is the result of the osmotic gradient and may force some patients to request other sclerosants.

Hypertonic dextrose/hypertonic saline (Sclerodex, Omega Laboratories Ltd, Montreal). Hypertonic saline and dextrose (HSD) is a mixture of dextrose 250 mg/ml, sodium chloride 100 mg/ml, propylene glycol 100 mg/ml, and phenethyl alcohol 8 mg/ml. HSD has been used predominately in Canada and is reported to result in less discomfort than hypertonic saline, although a slightly burning sensation can occur.[5] The lower saline concentration combined with the nonionic dextrose causes a hypertonic

Table 5-2 Relative Potency and Use of Sclerosing Solutions

Vein Diameter	Sclerosing Solution
<0.4mm	Hypertonic saline 11.7%
	Chromated glycerin 50%
	Polidocanol 0.25%
	Sodium tetradecyl sulfate 0.1%
	Chromated glycerin 100%
	Polidocanol 0.5%
	Polyiodide iodine 0.1%
	Sodium morrhuate 1%
	Ethanolamine oleate 2%
	Hypertonic dextrose and saline
0.6–2mm	Hypertonic dextrose and saline
	Sodium tetradecyl sulfate 0.2–0.3%
	Polidocanol 0.5–0.75%
	Polyiodide iodine 1.0%
	Hypertonic saline 23.4%
	Ethanolamine oleate 5%
	Sodium morrhuate 2.5%
3–5mm	Polidocanol 1–2%
	Sodium tetradecyl sulfate 0.5–1.0%
	Polyiodide iodine 2%
	Sodium morrhuate 5%
>5mm	Polidocanol 3–5%
Perforators	Sodium tetradecyl sulfate 2–3%
Saphenopopliteal & Saphenofemoral Junction	Polyiodide iodine 3–12%

(Modified from Goldman MP: Sclerotherapy Treatment of Varicose and Telangiectatic Leg Veins. St Louis, 1991, Mosby.)

injury without the intense, nerve-ending stimulation of pure HS. The higher viscosity probably allows increased contact time with the vessel wall before intravascular dilution of the osmotic gradient.

HSD is recommended for local treatment of small telangiectasia and venulectasia, with a total volume of injection not to exceed 10 ml per visit and 0.1 ml to 1.0 ml per injection site (Sclerodex prescribing information. J Dermatolog Surg Oncol 17:63-4 1991.) HSD use has resulted in fewer complications and less cutaneous necrosis than HS, but has a similar incidence of pigmentation compared with polidocanol and sodium tetradecyl sulfate.[6] An additional advantage is decreased

pain on injection. Allergenicity of the phenethyl alcohol component of HSD is possible, with a reported incidence of allergic reactions of 1/500.[5] Use in the United States awaits FDA approval.

Detergent Solutions

The detergents act as emulsifiers, causing dissolution of the endothelial cell membrane by the polar (hydrophilic) portion aligning with water molecules and the nonpolar (hydrophobic) portion inserting into the lipid cell membrane. This reaction occurs quickly compared with hyperosmotic injury. The "strength" of the detergent, and its capacity to cause lipid to be water soluble, determines the depth of injury. Once the endothelial cell layer disintegrates, the media and adventitia can be rapidly destroyed. This process is concentration dependent[7] and appears clinically to induce more inflammation than hyperosmotic injury (Fig. 5-1). The destructive effect of a detergent solution can spread far beyond the injection site, as dilution weakens, but does not negate a lipid solubilizing effect.

Sodium tetradecyl sulfate (Sotradecol, Wyeth-Ayerst Labs, Philadelphia; S.T.D. Injection, S.T.D. Pharmaceuticals, United Kingdom; Thromboject, Omega Labs, Montreal). Sodium tetradecyl sulfate (STS) is the most popular solution in the United States for treating large varicosities and is rapidly gaining acceptance for treatment of telangiectasia (Figs. 5-3 and 5-4). STS is a long-chain, fatty-acid salt with strong detergent properties and is a very effective sclerosing agent approved by the FDA since 1946. Its use reported occasionally by vascular surgeons since the 1960s[8-10] and described for telangiectasias in the 1970s,[11] STS has a possibly undeserved reputation of high incidence of postsclerosis pigmentation and the possibility of cutaneous necrosis even in the absence of recognized extravasation.[12] Cutaneous necrosis as high as 60-70% with 1% STS can be reduced to 3% by using 0.33% STS.[12] Rabbit-skin injection of 0.5% STS (0.1 ml) leads to dermal and epidermal necrosis.[13] Although noted to cause allergic reactions such as generalized urticaria, bronchospasm, anaphylactic shock, and even death, the actual incidence of allergic reactions is relatively low, estimated at 0.3%.[14, 15]

Interpretation of available data leads to recommendations of use of 0.1-0.2% for telangiectasias up to 1 mm, 0.2-0.5% in reticular veins or small varicosities (1-3 mm diameter), and 0.5-3% in larger varicosities related to major sites of valvular reflux. The maximum dosage per treatment session recommended in the package insert is 10 ml of 3% solution.

Polidocanol (POL) (Aethoxysklerol, Chemische Fabrik Kreussler & Co, Wiesbaden-Biebrich, West Germany; Aetoxisclerol, Laboratories Pharmaceutiques Dexo, Nanterre, France; Sclerovein, Resinag AG,

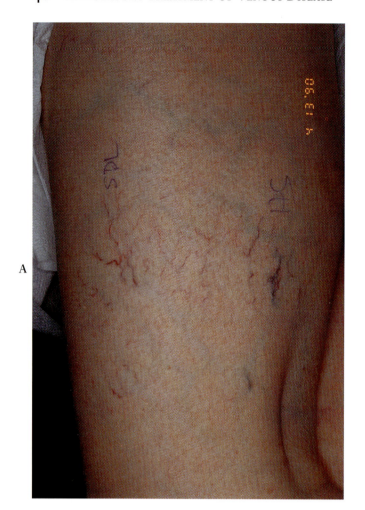

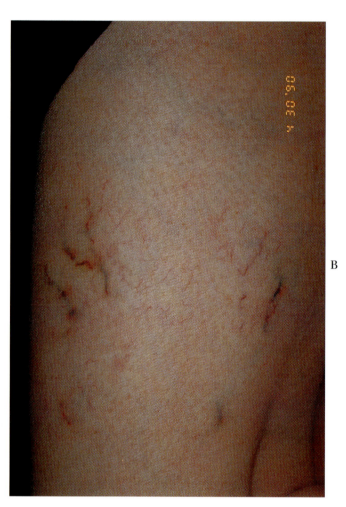

Fig. 5-1. Use of sclerosant higher than the minimal sclerosant concentration. **A,** A region on the lateral thigh treated with 0.2% STS (noted as SDL in photo) with an adjacent area treated with 23.4% HS (noted as HS). Immediate response showed marked urtication in both areas with much surrounding erythema. **B,** Two weeks later, hyperpigmentation is noted in both areas. This is probably the result of being higher than the minimal sclerosant concentration. For this patient the next treatment should consist of either 0.1% STS or 11.7% HS. Particular attention should also be paid to any sources of reflux into this region that could increase trapping of red blood cells. **C,** Another patient who has been treated for medial thigh venulectatic web. A reticular vein was treated with 0.5% STS, and the associated venulectases were treated with 0.1% STS. **D,** Two weeks later, hyperpigmentation appears in the venulectases. Repeat Doppler examination revealed continued reflux into the area. Repeat treatment of reticular vein with 0.5% STS caused resolution of the hyperpigmentation within six months.

Zurich, Switzerland). First used as a sclerosing agent in the late 1960s in Germany, POL is popular worldwide because of the painless injection and the extremely rare incidence of cutaneous necrosis with intradermal injection.[13, 16] POL is *not* approved by the FDA, and its use is presently prohibited in the United States unless authorized for phase III clinical trials. Until recently POL was thought to be the safest sclerosant, with an extremely low incidence of side effects. Recent reports of anaphylactic and other reactions place POL within the same safety range as STS.[17, 18]

In the dorsal rabbit ear vein model, 1% POL is equivalent to 0.5% STS and HS.[19] By extrapolating from several clinical studies, when used on human telangiectasia 0.5% POL appears equivalent to HS and 0.1%-0.2% STS. Lower concentrations of POL have demonstrated a lower incidence of hyperpigmentation than HS or STS.[4]

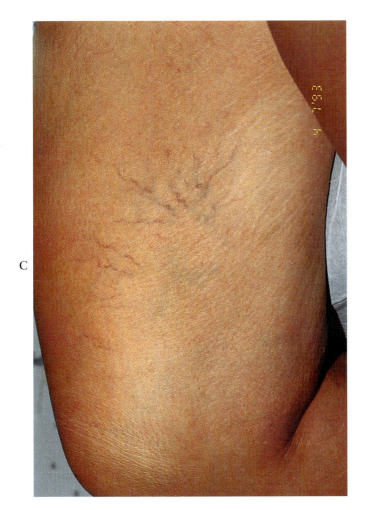 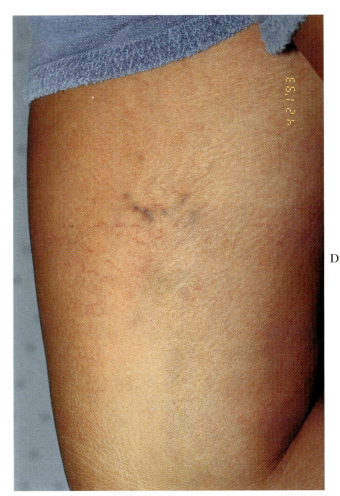

C   D

Fig. 5-1, cont'd. For legend see opposite page.

Sodium Morrhuate (Scleromate, Palisades Pharmaceuticals, Inc., Tenafly, N.J.) Sodium morrhuate (SM) is a 5% solution of the salts of saturated and unsaturated fatty acids in cod-liver oil. Approximately 10% of its fatty acid composition is unknown and routine use is limited by reports of fatalities secondary to anaphylaxis.[20, 21] This agent is used primarily for sclerosis of esophageal varices, but complications including allergic reactions are reported as high as 17-48%.[22] Of note is that there have been no reports of allergic reactions involving SM in recent medical literature. Although SM is approved by the FDA for the sclerosis of varicose veins, treating telangiectasias with SM is not recommended because of the caustic qualities and increased potential for cutaneous necrosis compared to other available solutions.

Ethanolamine oleate (Block Drug Co., Piscataway, N.J.). Ethanolamine oleate (EO) is a synthetic mixture of ethanolamine and oleic acid. The oleic acid component is responsible for inflammation. Although EO is mainly used in this country for sclerosis of esophageal varices, it is commonly used in Australia for sclerotherapy of varicose veins. Anaphylactic shock has been reported following injection in a number of patients.[23, 24] Generalized urticaria occurred in about 1/400 patients and cleared with antihistamines.[25]

Corrosive agents

These agents, including a diverse roup of substances from alcohols to salts to heavy metals, are believed to work by protein denaturation. They act quickly, interact, and disrupt proteins indiscriminately, but are rapidly consumed in the process. Therefore the effect is limited more to the actual injection site compared with detergent sclerosants. This is a distinct advantage when larger vessels are treated and injury must be limited to a small segment. The destruction depth is determined by the potency of caustic effect; a strong solution can cause full thickness vessel destruction within seconds, whereas another agent's caustic effect may be weak enough to cause only an extremely mild injury. The two extremes are illustrated by glycerin and polyiodide iodine. Using corrosive agents in the United States lacks FDA approval at this time.

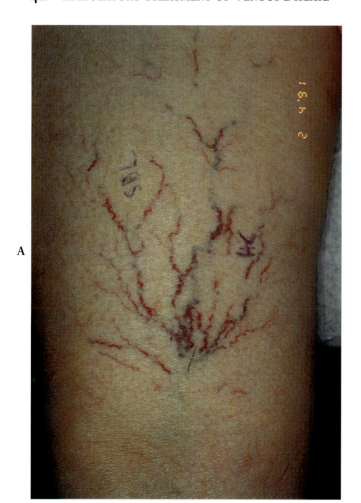

A

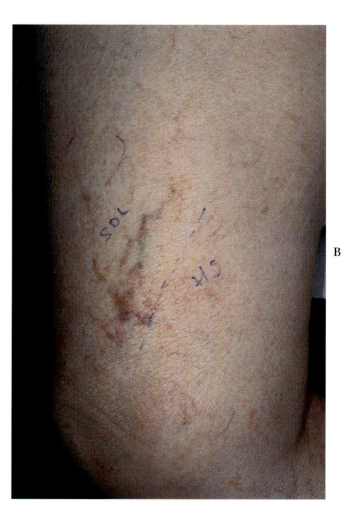

B

Fig. 5-2. Comparison of response to different classes of sclerosing solutions in venulectases. **A,** Medial thigh venulectatic web is associated with a reticular vein arising medial to the patella. The dorsal half was treated with 0.2% STS (noted as SDL), and the ventral half was treated with 23.4% HS. The immediate response was much greater inflammation with STS. The reticular vein (not shown) was treated simultaneously with 0.5% STS. **B,** Three months posttreatment photograph shows persistence of marked hyperpigmentation with 0.2% STS and complete resolution with 23.4% HS. For this patient, the hyperosmotic solution caused marked decreased inflammation with less perivascular leakage of red blood cells than the detergent solution. Perhaps a trial of 0.1% STS would yield similar results to the use of 23.4% HS, although some patients have inflammatory responses with detergent solutions even at very low concentrations. The region of the lower medial thigh also seems to be more susceptible to side effects of telangiectatic matting and hyperpigmentation. The most productive course for continuing treatment in this patient would be to use 23.4% HS for the remaining venulectatic webs.

Polyiodide iodine (Varigloban, Chemische Fabrik Kreussler & Co, Wiesbaden-Biebrich, West Germany; Variglobin, Globopharm, Switzerland; Sclerodine, Omega, Montreal). Polyiodide (PII) is a stabilized water solution of iodide ions, sodium iodine, and benzyl alcohol. The active sclerosing ingredient is iodine with sodium and potassium, which increases its water solubility. After injection of PII, the endothelium is destroyed within seconds; the corrosive agent can then penetrate further and diffuse into deeper layers of the vessel wall, causing ongoing destruction. Binding to blood components neutralizes PII within a few seconds, thus diminishing its sclerosing effect within a few centimeters.[26] PII is reserved for large varicosities with major reflux. Paravenous injections produce extensive tissue necrosis. Fortunately, PII is painful when injected outside a vein so that improper injection technique is immediately apparent. To enhance sclerosing power

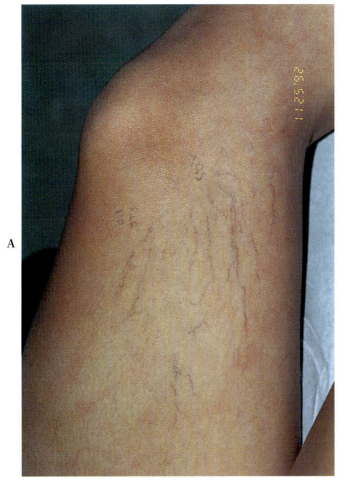

A

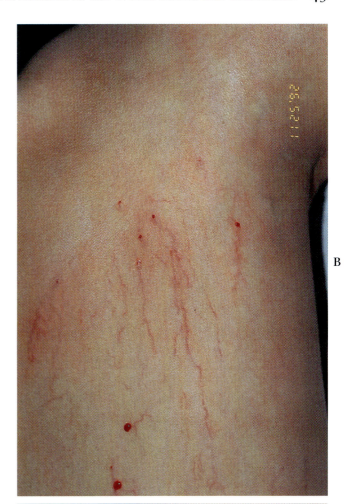

B

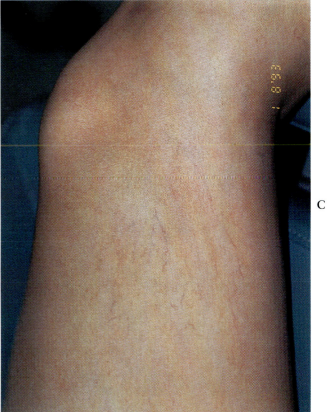

C

Fig. 5-3.   Comparison of hyperosmotic and detergent sclerosing solutions for a telangiectatic web. **A,** Adjacent areas of telangiectatic webs on the lateral thigh that were treated simultaneously with 0.1% STS and hypertonic saline and dextrose (abbreviated in the photo as SDX, new abbreviation HSD). **B,** Minutes after injection, the area treated with STS shows more signs of inflammation with marked urtication and total disruption of telangiectasia, but no extravasation of red blood cells. The region treated with HSD shows slight edema with visible margins of vessels well preserved. **C,** Approximately 6 weeks later the results are similar. Most originally treated telangiectasias have resolved or have recanalized with a much smaller diameter. A few telangiectasia that were not injected with any sclerosing solution (in between the two treatment regions) show no improvement at all. In this patient, both sclerosing solutions were administered as the minimal sclerosant concentration, that is, effective sclerosis with a minimum number of side effects. Treatment of other regions with similar caliber telangiectasias would probably be effective with either solution.

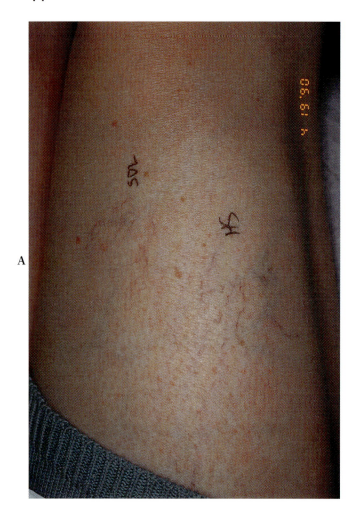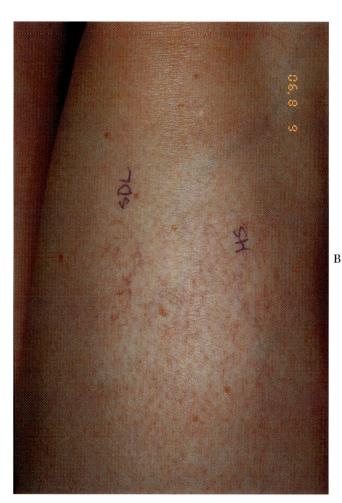

Fig. 5-4. Incomplete resolution below the minimal sclerosant concentration. **A,** The right lateral thigh is shown with associated lateral venous system reticular vein. In this patient the reticular vein was not treated at the same time as the telangiectasia. One telangiectatic web is treated with 0.1% STS (noted as SDL) and a nearby web is treated with 23.4% HS. **B,** One month later the region treated with HS has resolved completely. Some residual telangiectasia remain at the site of STS injection. The untreated reticular vein remains as well. For this patient the MSC for STS is probably slightly higher than 0.1%. Many other factors are involved, however, such as the volume and pressure of injection and the presence of reflux from a larger vein into the region. In this patient these factors were equalized as much as possible with 0.1 ml of each solution and identical injection pressure. The treated telangiectasias would probably recur within a year if reflux from the associated reticular vein(s) was not eliminated.

and minimize nonspecific damage, the concentration of solution is increased, not the volume.

Chromated Glycerin, 72% (Chromex, Omega Laboratories, Montreal, Quebec) Chromated Glycerin, 72% (CGLY) is a polyalcohol with very mild corrosive activity. The activity of glycerin is potentiated slightly by the addition of a chromium salt. CGLY provokes endothelial lesions without desquamation of endothelial cells in plaques.[1] Its clinical efficacy has been shown to be dose dependent with a very low incidence

of adverse sequelae.[27] In the dorsal rabbit ear vein,[28] undiluted CGLY appears equivalent in potency to 0.25% POL. The relatively weak sclerosing power of CGLY corresponds with a low incidence of pigmentation and cutaneous necrosis.[29] Slight disadvantages of CGLY include its high viscosity and slight local pain with injection. These drawbacks can be partially overcome by dilution with 1% lidocaine without epinephrine. Hypersensitivity is very rare.[30]

COMPARISON OF SCLEROSING SOLUTIONS BY MOST COMMON SIDE EFFECTS

Hyperpigmentation

The general incidence of hyperpigmentation ranges from 10-30% in patients treated with hypertonic saline (HS),[2, 31-34] and 10.7%[35] to 30%[31, 36] in patients treated with polidocanol (POL). Telangiectasias treated with 1% POL have been reported to yield a higher incidence of hyperpigmentation than HS or 0.5% POL[37] (Fig. 5-5). With higher concentrations of sodium tetradecyl sulfate (STS), hyperpigmentation incidence is 30%[38] to 80%,[11] although using 0.1% STS concentration lowers the incidence to 11%.[2] Although certain sclerosing solutions theoretically have lower risks of causing pigmentation, one can conclude that the concentration of a particular solution plays a major role. Other factors such as technique, injection pressures, and degree of venous hypertension must also be considered.

Cloutier and Sansoucy[39] and Tournay[38] state that STS has the highest incidence of pigmentation amongst sclerosing solutions. Although Goldman[40] and Duffy[31] noted a similar incidence of pigmentation between HS and STS, Weiss and Weiss noted a 10.8% incidence of pigmentation with HS compared to a 30.7% incidence with 1% POL for telangiectasia[37] and have also reported a slightly higher incidence of hyperpigmentation with STS compared with HS.[41]

Sclerosing solutions reported to have the lowest incidence of postsclerotherapy pigmentation are chemical irritants such as chromated glycerin (CG).[29, 37, 39, 42-46] A retrospective study of 135 patients investigated whether replacing POL with CG would lower the incidence of pigmentation.[47] CG was used as the initial sclerosing agent; when CG caused a strong inflammatory reaction, patients were switched to POL. Hyperpigmentation only developed in 8% of CG-treated patients and in none of the POL-treated patients. This trial argues for using preliminary sclerotherapy tests with different classes of sclerosing solutions before proceeding with definitive treatment.

In addition to type of sclerosing solution, concentration can also affect the pigmentation development. Norris, Carlin, and Ratz observed an increased incidence of pigmentation (60%) in telangiectasias treated with 1% POL compared with 0.5% POL (20%).[48] Weiss and Weiss noted a similar decrease in pigmentation between 1% POL (30.7%) and 0.5% POL (10%).[37] High concentrations of sclerosing solutions or using extremely caustic agents in small-diameter vessels probably increases perivascular inflammation with accompanying cutaneous red blood cell leakage and deposition.

Telangiectatic matting

As with hyperpigmentation, limiting the amount of inflammation associated with sclerotherapy of a given vessel diameter will theoretically reduce the incidence of telangiectatic matting (TM). This can be achieved by using the minimal sclerosant concentration (MSC) for a given vessel diameter and limiting the quantity of sclerosant used at a given injection site, thus producing less endothelial damage[4] (Fig. 5-6). Corroborating this theory, a study of 10 patients who developed TM with injection of POL 1% into vessels less than 1 mm in diameter found that the patients did not develop further areas of TM when POL 0.5% was used.[37] Further support of this theory are the studies of Ouvry and Davy[49] and Mantse[6] who noted a decreased incidence of TM when injection pressures and extent of dispersion of sclerosing solution were limited to 1 cm with each injection.

Necrosis

POL appears experimentally to be minimally toxic to subcutaneous tissue. Intradermal POL 0.5% is even used to treat telangiectatic leg veins smaller than the diameter of a 30-gauge needle with no evidence of cutaneous necrosis.[50, 51] However, POL in sufficient concentration has been reported to cause necrosis.[20, 50] CG solutions have not been reported to produce cutaneous necrosis with extravasation. As mentioned, any sclerosant in sufficient concentration and volume

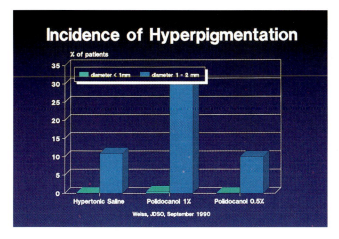

Fig. 5-5. Relative Incidence of Hyperpigmentation. Hyperpigmentation is relatively rare in vessels below 1mm in diameter. Reducing POL concentration greatly reduces the incidence of hyperpigmentation. (From Weiss RA, Weiss MA: Incidence of side effects in the treatment of telangiectasias by compression sclerotherapy: hypertonic saline vs. polidocanol, J Dermatol Surg Oncol 16:800–804, 1990.)

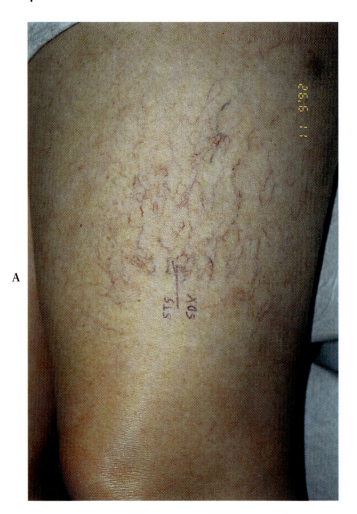 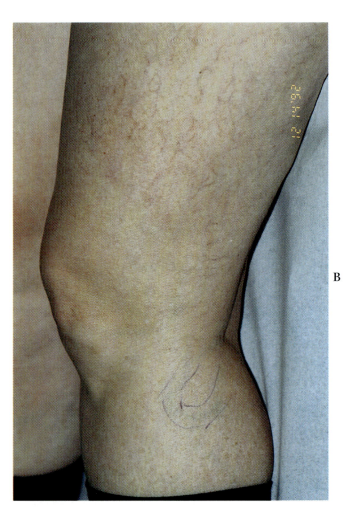

Fig. 5-6.   Appearance of telangiectatic matting with minimal sclerosant concentration. **A,** The lateral thigh of telangiectatic web was treated fractionally with 0.1% STS and HSD (noted as SDX). The line marked on the skin shows the division between the two solutions. **B,** Results at 1 month: There is equal resolution on the thigh with excellent response. Some telangiectatic matting is noted with both solutions. Repeat physical and Doppler examination reveals a large reticular vein effecting reflux into this region (outlined in blue pen). This was subsequently treated with 0.5% STS (1 cc total). The reticular vein and associated telangiectatic matting resolved within 3 months posttreatment.

injected superficially enough to minimize rapid dissolution can induce necrosis.

◼ CONCLUSIONS

An experienced phlebologist can use any of the wide variety of sclerosants discussed here. (Table 5-3) Physicians in the United States are limited in their choice at this time, but can hopefully look forward to FDA approval of polidocanol within a reasonable period. Even so, with clear understanding of the properties of hypertonic saline and sodium tetradecyl sulfate, a U.S. physician can offer excellent treatment of both telangiectasias and varicose veins. There is no single

ideal agent for sclerotherapy; physicians must gain experience with those agents and their concentrations best suited for the clinical situation presented by an individual patient.

◼ REFERENCES

1. Imhoff E, Stemmer R: Classification and mechanism of action of sclerosing agents. Bull de la Soc Fran de Phlebol 22:143-148, 1969.

2. Weiss RA, Weiss MA: Resolution of pain associated with varicose and telangiectatic leg veins after compression sclerotherapy. J Dermatol Surg Oncol 16:333-336, 1990.

TABLE 5-3 Rapid Guide for Selection of Sclerosing Solution by Vessel Type*

Vessel	Solution, Concentration	Volume (per region)
Telangiectatic matting (after previous treatment)	Chromated glycerin, diluted by 50%	0.1–0.2 ml
Telangiectasia (up to 1 mm)	**Hypertonic saline, 11.7%** **Sodium tetradecyl sulfate, 0.1%** Hypertonic saline and dextrose, Chromated glycerin, 50% Polidocanol, 0.25%	0.1–0.3 ml
Venulectasia (1–2 mm)	**Hypertonic saline, 11.7%–23.4%** **Sodium tetradecyl sulfate, 0.1–0.25%** Hypertonic saline 10% and dextrose, 25% (Sclerodex) Chromated glycerin, 100% Polidocanol, 0.5%	0.2–0.5 ml
Reticular veins (2–4 mm - subcutaneous blue veins)	**Hypertonic saline, 23.4%** **Sodium tetradecyl sulfate, 0.33–0.5%** **Sodium morrhuate, 2.5%** Polidocanol, 1.0% Polyiodide iodine, 0.3–1.0%	0.5 ml (may increase to 1 ml if filling of reticular vein is observed)
Nonsaphenous varicose veins (3–8mm)	**Sodium tetradecyl sulfate, 0.5–1.0%** **Sodium morrhuate, 5%** Polidocanol, 1.0–3.0% Polyiodide iodine, 1.0–2.0%	0.5 ml (may increase to 1 ml per injection site in large capacity vein, except for polyiodide)
Saphenous varicose trunks (usually >5mm)	**Sodium tetradecyl sulfate, 1.0–3.0%** Polidocanol, 3.0–5.0% Polyiodide iodine, 2.0–6.0% (rarely to 12%)	0.5 ml (low-volume injection critical at high concentrations)

* Solutions approved by US FDA in bold

3. Sadick NS: Treatment of varicose and telangiectatic leg veins with hypertonic saline: a comparative study of heparin and saline. J Dermatol Surg Oncol 16:24-28, 1990.

4. Sadick NS: Sclerotherapy of varicose and telangiectatic leg veins. Minimal sclerosant concentration of hypertonic saline and its relationship to vessel diameter [see comments]. J Dermatol Surg Oncol 17:65-70, 1991.

5. Mantse L: A mild sclerosing agent for telangiectasias [letter]. J Dermatol Surg Oncol 11:855, 1985.

6. Mantse L: More on spider veins [letter]. J Dermatol Surg Oncol 12:1022-1023, 1986.

7. Rotter SM, Weiss RA: Human saphenous vein in vitro model for studying the action of sclerosing solutions. J Dermatol Surg Oncol 19:59-62, 1993.

8. Hobbs JT: Surgery and sclerotherapy in the treatment of varicose veins: a random trial. Arch Surg 109:793-796, 1974.

9. Hobbs JT: The treatment of varicose veins: a random trial of injection/compression versus surgery. Br J Surg 55:777-780, 1968.

10. Fegan WG: Continuous compression technique of injecting varicose veins. Lancet 2:109-112, 1963.

11. Tretbar LL: Spider angiomata: treatment with sclerosant injections. J Kansas Med Soc 79:198-200, 1978.

12. Tretbar LL: Injection sclerotherapy for spider telangiectasias: a 20-year experience with sodium tetradecyl sulfate. J Dermatol Surg Oncol 15:223-225, 1989.

13. Goldman MP, Kaplan RP, Oki LN, et al.: Extravascular effects of sclerosants in rabbit skin: A clinical and histologic examination. J Dermatol Surg Oncol 12: 1085-1088, 1986.

14. Passas H: One case of tetradecyl-sodium sulfate allergy with general symptoms. Soc Fran de Phlebol 25:19, 1972.

15. Goldman MP, Bennet RG: Treatment of telangiectasia: a review. J Am Acad Dermatol 17:167-182, 1987.

16. Eichenberger H: Results of phlebosclerosation with hydroxypolyethoxydodecane. Zentralbl Phlebol 8:181-183, 1969.

17. Stricker BHC, Van Oijen JA, Kroon C, Ovink AHOD: Anafylaxie na gebruik van polidocanol [Anaphylaxis after use of polidocanol]. Ned Tijdschr Geneeskd 134:240-242, 1990.

18. Feied CF, Jackson JJ, Bren TS, Bond OB, Fernando CE, Young VCY, Hashemiyoon RB: Allergic reactions to polidocanol for vein sclerosis: two case reports. J Dermatol Surg Oncol 20:466-468, 1994.

19. Goldman MP, Kaplan RP, Oki LN, et al.: Sclerosing agents in the treatment of telangiectasia: comparison of the clinical and histologic effects of intravascular polidocanol, sodium tetradecyl sulfate, and hypertonic saline in the dorsal rabbit ear vein model. Arch Dermatol 123: 1196-1201, 1987.

20. Goldman MP: Sclerotherapy: Treatment of varicose and telangiectatic leg veins. St Louis, 1991, Mosby, 239-246.

21. Lewis KM: Anaphylaxis due to sodium morrhuate. JAMA 107:1298-1299, 1936.

22. Sarin SK, Kumar A: Sclerosants for variceal sclerotherapy: a critical appraisal. Am J Gastroenterol 85: 641-649, 1990.

23. Foote RR: Severe reaction to monoethanolamine oleate. Lancet 2:390-391, 1944.

24. Hughes RW, Jr., et al.: Endoscopic variceal sclerosis: a one-year experience. Gastrointest Endosc 28:62-68, 1982.

25. Reid RG, Rothnie NG: Treatment of varicose veins by compression sclerotherapy. Br J Surg 55:889-895, 1968.

26. Wenner L: Anwendung einer mit athylalkohol modifizierten polijodidjonenlosung bei skleroseresistenten varizen. Vasa 12:190-192, 1983.

27. Ouvry PA, Davy A: The sclerotherapy of telangiectasia. Phlebol 35:349-359, 1982.

28. Martin DE, Goldman MP: A comparison of sclerosing agents: clinical and histologic effects of intravascular sodium tetradecyl sulfate and chromated glycerine in the dorsal rabbit ear vein. J Dermatol Surg Oncol 16:18-22, 1990.

29. Nebot F: Quelques points tecniques sur le traitement des varicosites et des telangiectasies. Phlebol 21:133-135, 1968.

30. Ouvry P, Arlaud R: Le traitement sclerosant des telangiectasies des membres inferieurs. Phlebol 32:365-370, 1979.

31. Duffy DM: Small vessel sclerotherapy: an overview. Adv Dermatol 3:221-242, 1988.

32. Alderman DB: Surgery and sclerotherapy in the treatment of varicose veins. Conn Med 39:467-471, 1975.

33. Bodian EL: Techniques of sclerotherapy for sunburst venous blemishes. J Dermatol Surg Oncol 11:696-704, 1985.

34. Alderman DB: Therapy for essential cutaneous telangiectasias. Postgrad Med 61:91-95, 1977.

35. Cacciatore E: [Experience with Atoxisclerol in sclerotherapy]. Minerva Cardioangiol 27:255-262, 1979.

36. Goldman PM: Sclerotherapy for superficial venules and telangiectasias of the lower extremities. Dermatol Clin 5:369-379, 1987.

37. Weiss RA, Weiss MA: Incidence of side effects in the treatment of telangiectasias by compression sclerotherapy: hypertonic saline vs. polidocanol. J Dermatol Surg Oncol 16:800-804, 1990.

38. Tournay PR: Traitment sclerosant des tres fines varicosites intra ou saous-dermiques. [Sclerosing treatment of very fine intra or subdermal varicosities]. Soc Fran de Phlebol 19:235-241, 1966.

39. Cloutier G, Sansoucy H: Le traitement des varices des membres inferieurs par les injections sclerosantes. L'Union Medicale du Canada 104:1854-1863, 1975.

40. Goldman MP, Kaplan RP, Duffy DM: Postsclerotherapy hyperpigmentation: a histologic evaluation. J Dermatol Surg Oncol 13:547-550, 1987.

41. Weiss MA, Weiss RA: Efficacy and side effects of 0.1% sodium tetradecyl sulfate in compression sclerotherapy of telangiectasias: comparison to 1% polidocanol and hypertonic saline. J Dermatol Surg Oncol 17:90-91 (Abstract), 1991.

42. Georgiev M: Postsclerotherapy hyperpigmentations: a one-year follow-up. J Dermatol Surg Oncol 16:608-610, 1990.

43. Hutinel B: Esthetique dans les scleroses de varices et traitement des varicosites. La Vie Medicale 20:1739-1743, 1978.

44. Landart J: Traitement medical des varices des membres inferieurs. La Revue du Practician 26:2491-2494, 1976.

45. Tournay R, Caille JP, Chatard H, et al.: La sclerose des varices. Paris: 1980, Expansion Scientifique.

46. Lucchi M, Bilancini S: Sclerotherapy of telangiectasia (English abstract). Minerva Angiol 15:31, 1990.

47. Georgiev M: Postsclerotherapy hyperpigmentations: chromated glycerin as a screen for patients at risk (a retrospective study). J Dermatol Surg Oncol 19:649-652, 1993.

48. Norris MJ, Carlin MC, Ratz JL: Treatment of essential telangiectasia: effects of increasing concentrations of polidocanol. J Am Acad Dermatol 20:683-689, 1989.

49. Ouvry P, Davy A: Le traitement sclerosant des telangiectasies des membres inferieurs. Phlebol 35:349-355, 1982.

50. Jaquier JJ, Loretan RM: Clinical trials of a new sclerosing agent, aethoxysklerol. Soc Fran de Phlebol 22: 383-385, 1969.

51. Hoffer AE: Aethoxysklerol (Kreussler) in the treatment of varices. Minn Cardioang 20:601-604, 1972.

6

SCLEROTHERAPY OF RETICULAR VEINS

Helane S. Fronek

The aim of sclerotherapy of telangiectasias is the disappearance of the treated veins and the symptoms caused by them. In many cases, this occurs quite predictably, yet in others the veins seem to be "resistant" or rapidly recur after initially disappearing. Although these treatment failures can be the result of an inadequate concentration of sclerosant or poor technique, several recent publications have presented evidence that this treatment failure may be due, at least in part, to the failure to recognize and treat another system of connected veins.[1-4] These veins, alternately called minor varicose veins, feeding veins, or reticular veins, are 1 to 4 mm in diameter, located parallel to the skin surface and just subcutaneous and appear green or blue to the observer. With duplex ultrasound examinations, Somjen and associates found that 89% of patients with thigh telangiectasias had reticular vein incompetence close to the telangiectasias.[3] These reticular veins communicated frequently with each other, forming an intricate network. Of equal importance was his finding that in seven legs without telangiectasias, no subcutaneous venous incompetence could be found. Weiss and Weiss, using continuous-wave Doppler, found the coexistence of incompetent reticular veins in 88% of patients with thigh telangiectasias.[4] Thus, it is likely that the development of incompetence in this network of subcutaneous vessels is important in telangiectatic vein formation and that correcting this incompetence can aid in the disappearance of the secondary telangiectasias.

Albanese speculated that some of these incompetent reticular venous networks, especially those along the lateral aspect of the leg, might be remnants of the embryonic venous system.[5] During embryonic development, the lesser saphenous vein is present superficially in both the calf and thigh, connected to a rudimentary deep venous system by small perforating veins. As the deep venous system becomes dominant, the lesser saphenous vein disappears above the knee. In some people, this superficial vein and its connecting perforating veins do not completely involute, and the result is what Albanese termed the lateral subdermic venous system (Fig. 6-1). With progressive weakening of the vessel wall or the transmission of an elevated pressure through the incompetent perforating veins, the reticular veins can become enlarged.[6] Also, it is now known that veins from patients who develop varicosities have a different chemical composition.[7] It is, therefore, probable that the reticular veins in these people are more capable of dilating under normal gravitational and hydrostatic pressures and will thus gradually enlarge. This enlargement is often the source of symptoms such as heaviness, aching, burning, itching, cramping, and pain and can also lead to cosmetically disturbing or symptomatic telangiectasias.

■ EXAMINATION

Several methods can be used to determine the presence and intensity of reflux in reticular veins. Somjen[3] used duplex ultrasonography which, although most revealing, is certainly more than what is required to evaluate and treat most patients. Weiss and Weiss advocate continuous-wave Doppler to determine reflux in suspicious reticular veins as well as to determine the loudest site of reflux, which they feel corresponds to the site of an incompetent perforating vein.[1,4] This site, usually just distal to the lateral femoral condyle, is where they initiate treatment.

In practice, any visible reticular vein underlying a cluster or web of telangiectasias should be treated before or at the same time as the overlying telangiectasias (Fig. 6-2). Somjen found that almost all reticular veins 2.5 mm or larger in diameter were incompetent.[3] Also,

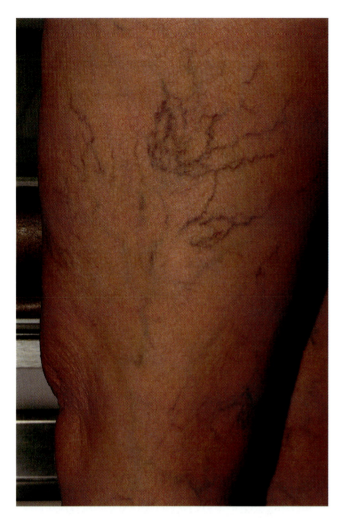

Fig. 6-1.   The lateral subdermic venous system is commonly visible as reticular veins with overlying telangiectasias.

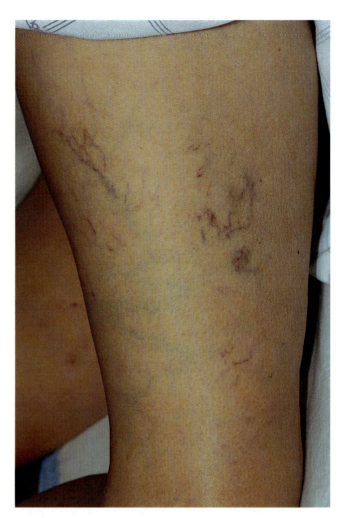

Fig. 6-2.   Any visible reticular vein underlying a cluster or web of telangiectasias should be treated before or at the same time as the overlying veins.

by recalling the distribution of the lateral subdermic venous system, one would also treat any visible reticular vein on the lateral thigh or calf along its entire course if lateral thigh telangiectasias are present. If in doubt, continuous-wave Doppler can certainly be employed to test for reflux. By repeatedly compressing the calf or simply the vein distal to the Doppler probe while the patient stands, reflux is easily heard within an incompetent reticular vein.

TREATMENT

After careful observation of the venous patterns with the patient standing, I will frequently ask the patient to lie down so that I can be sure that all of the incompetent reticular veins are clearly visible. In general, no premarking of the skin is necessary, as these veins are usually visible from the skin surface. However, if a reticular vein seen with the patient standing is no longer clearly visible when he lies down, I will ask the patient to stand again so that I can mark the vein. All injections are performed with the patient lying down and the veins to be treated fully visible. A 3 cc disposable syringe is filled with the appropriate solution (see Table 6-1) and is connected to a 30 Ga needle (Air-tite of Virginia, Inc.). I like to bend the needle just distal to the hub so that the bevel will face the skin surface (Fig. 6-3). It does not matter whether the bevel is down (as I

TABLE 6-1   Sclerosants Appropriate for Injection of Reticular Veins

Sodium tetradecyl sulfate	0.3–0.6%
Hypertonic saline	23.4%
Polidocanol	0.75–1.5%
Polyiodinated iodine	1%

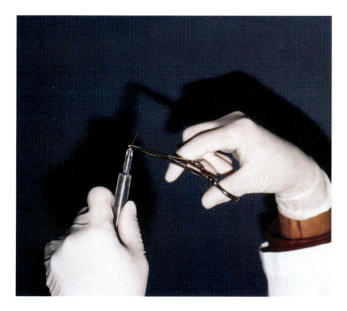

Fig. 6-3. The needle is bent approximately 20 degrees, just distal to the hub, to facilitate cannulation of the vein.

use it) or up, but the needle should be angled slightly (about 20 degrees) to allow one to advance it parallel to the skin surface after the skin has been punctured. With experience, one can use two quick motions to enter the vein—the first to pierce the skin, and the second to cannulate the vein (Fig. 6-4). Entry into the vein is felt as a distinct pop, or sudden decrease in resistance, although this perception is gained only after some experience. Until then it is advisable to pierce the skin and then gradually advance the needle while pulling back gently on the plunger of the syringe. As soon as blood is seen in the hub of the needle the sclerosant can be injected. Generally, not more than 0.5 ml of sclerosant should be injected at any site, even though several milliliters can easily be needed to fill an entire vein. If resistance to injection occurs or if the vein goes into spasm, the needle is withdrawn and another injection is begun along the course of the vein. Injections can be done at variable intervals; approximately every 3 to 8 cm is common. With some solutions, the patient may experience burning or stinging in the treated area. Reassurance that this sensation will resolve in 5 to 10 minutes is generally the only intervention required. However, if the patient is too uncomfortable, firm manual compression of the vein or the tight application of an Ace bandage will usually relieve the pain quite promptly.

After the entire leg has been treated, I apply Dermafit, a cotton stockinette available in several diameters, over the leg (Fig. 6-5). Over very protuberant reticular veins or those on the posterior aspect of the thigh or popliteal fossa I tape ½" foam pads cut to the length of the treated vein and beveled so that the central area is highest. Over this I place a class 2 graduated compression stocking (Fig. 6-6). This is worn con-

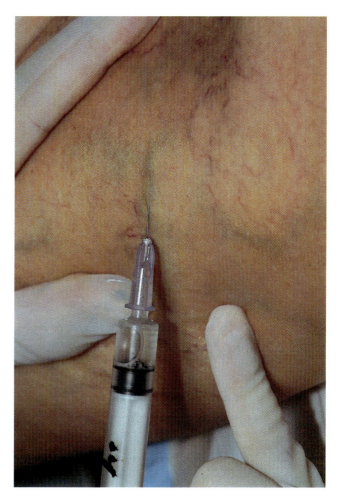

Fig. 6-4. Traction on the skin allows quick entry of the needle into the skin, directly over the reticular vein. A second motion is used to cannulate the vein.

tinuously for one week. If the patient is particularly intolerant of this compression, the stocking may be removed nightly starting with the second night, but worn during the day for the full week.

■ SIDE EFFECTS

Intravascular thrombi are common and should be evacuated as aggressively as possible to decrease the frequency and intensity of hyperpigmentation, a side effect that usually disappears within 6 to 12 months following treatment (Fig. 6-7, A and B). Until they are evacuated these thrombi can be the source of tender lumps over the treated veins. After local anesthesia has been achieved, the clot can be expressed through a 20-gauge needle puncture (Fig. 6-8, A and B). Compression need not be worn following this procedure, unless a large amount has been removed. Repeated evacuation of clot, usually at weekly intervals, is necessary in the rare patient.

A 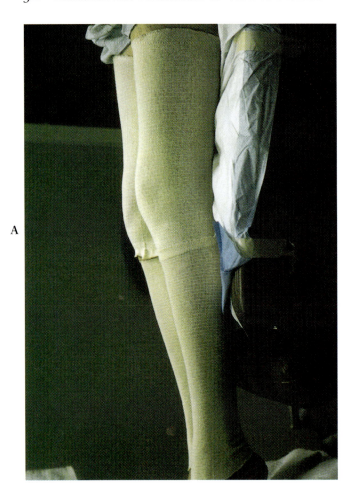 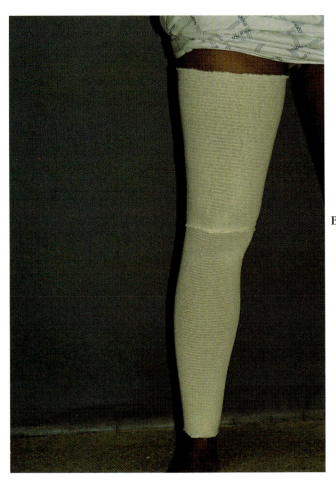 B

Fig. 6-5. Dermafit, a cotton stockinette is applied to the leg to provide initial compression, aid in hemostasis, and protect the stocking from blood which can ooze from the injection sites for several minutes. The Dermafit may later be pulled out by the patient to prevent chafing behind the knee, resulting from bunching of the fabric in this area.

The initial bruising will generally disappear within two weeks, but can recur after the thrombi removal (Fig. 6-9). Telangiectatic matting is possible, although not frequent. In those rare cases where the matting does not resolve with time, sclerotherapy using 11.7% to 15.9% saline solution or 0.1% to 0.4% Sotradecol or flash lamp pumped pulsed-dye laser treatment can be attempted.

■ PITFALLS

The most difficult aspect of reticular vein injections is finding the depth of the vein. Generally, by placing the needle under the skin directly overlying the vein and then advancing the needle while aspirating, one can tell when the needle has entered the vein. With experience, this may no longer be necessary. An intravas-cular position of the needle can be felt and the displacement of blood by the sclerosant can readily be appreciated once injection is begun (Fig. 6-10A to C).

The other common difficulty encountered is determining which reticular veins need to be treated. As mentioned previously, any reticular vein lying under a cluster of telangiectasis should be treated. Further, any reticular vein 2.5 mm or more in diameter in the vicinity of telangiectasias should be considered incompetent. Lastly, where a doubt exists, continuous-wave Doppler examination can be used to determine the status of the vein in question.

Injecting reticular veins is usually a very gratifying procedure, as it is followed by significant symptom alleviation as well as cosmetic improvement. Further, it will significantly improve long-term results of sclerotherapy of telangiectasias.

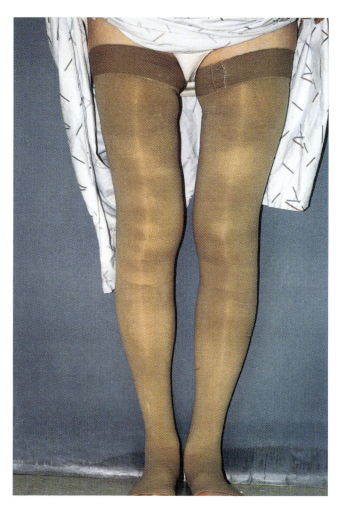

Fig. 6-6. A graduated, 30-40 mmHg compression stocking is worn for 3-7 days, depending on the size and number of veins being treated.

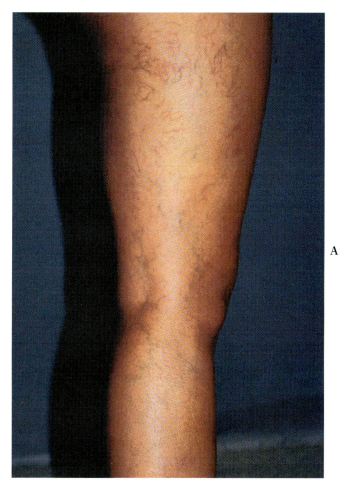

A

Fig. 6-7. Temporary pigmentation resulting from the treatment of reticular veins is common. This 40-year-old woman came for treatment of spider veins that had developed with her pregnancies and were associated with aching in her leg. **A,** Two months after the reticular vein alone was injected with 0.4% sodium tetradecyl sulfate, pigmentation was noted.

—Continued.

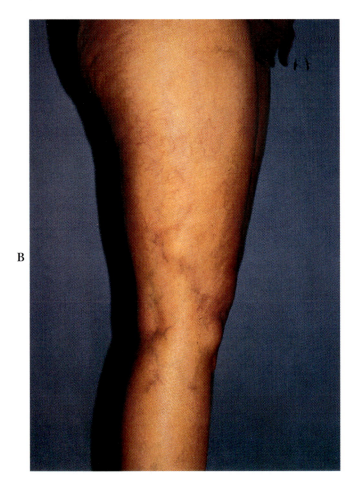

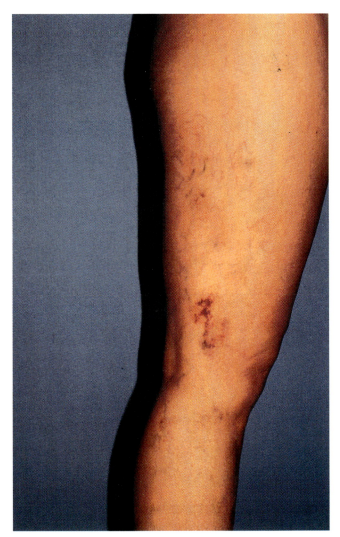

Fig. 6-7, cont'd. **B,** A marked reduction in the density of telangiectasias can also be seen. The pigmentation resolved after 10 months.

Fig. 6-9. Bruising is normal for several weeks after treatment and can recur after thrombi are removed.

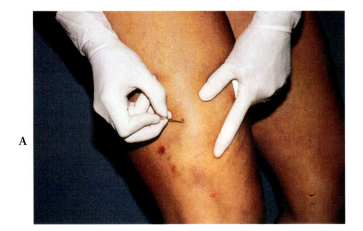

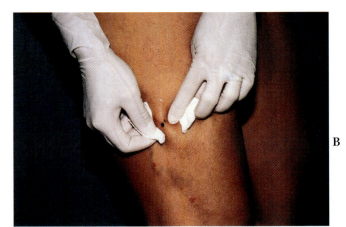

Fig. 6-8. Thrombi can frequently be removed from tender, firm areas. **A,** Punctures are made using a 20-gauge needle or the tip of a #11 scalpel. **B,** The thrombus is expressed by "milking" it out of the vein in both directions.

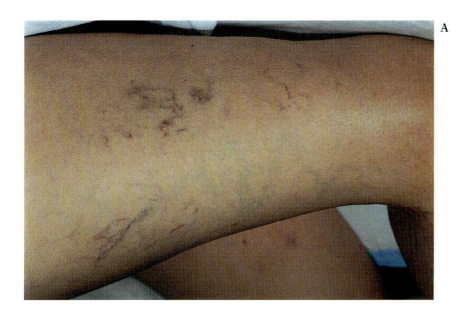

A

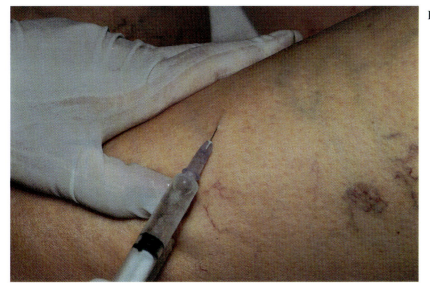

B

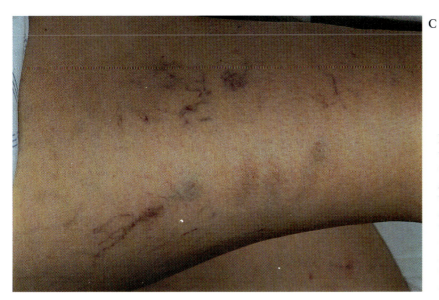

C

Fig. 6-10. Successful cannulation of reticular veins is readily apparent. Reticular veins underlying clusters of telangiectasias are targeted for injection. **A,** An intravascular position of the needle is appreciated by the immediate disappearance of the vein being treated. **B,** Several minutes after injection, urtication, induration, and erythema can be noted along the course of the treated vein. **C,** This can be associated with stinging or itching that stops within minutes.

■ REFERENCES

1. Weiss RA and Weiss MA: Doppler ultrasound findings in reticular veins of the thighs, J Dermatol Surg Oncol 18:62, 1992.

2. Bohler-Sommeregger K, Karnel F, and Schuller-Petrovic S: Do telangiectasias communicate with the deep venous system? J Dermatol Surg Oncol 18:403, 1993.

3. Somjen GM, Ziegenbein R, Johnson AH, and Royle JP: Anatomical examination of leg telangiectases with duplex scanning, J Dermatol Surg Oncol 19:940, 1993.

4. Weiss RA and Weiss MA: Doppler ultrasound findings in reticular veins of the thigh subdermic lateral venous system and implications for sclerotherapy, J Dermatol Surg Oncol 19:947, 1993.

5. Albanese AR, Albanese AM, and Albanese EF: The lateral subdermic venous system of the legs, Vasc Surg 3:81, 1969.

6. Weiss RA and Weiss MA: Painful telangiectasias: diagnosis and treatment. In: Began JJ and Goldman MP, editors: Varicose veins and telangiectasias. St Louis, 1993, Quality Medical Publishing, 389-406.

7. Browse NL, Burnand KG, and Lea TM: Diseases of the veins. London, 1988, Edward Arnold.

7

Injection Compression Sclerotherapy of Spider Telangiectasia and Small Varicose Veins

John R. Pfeifer

Although injection of cutaneous spider veins or telangiectasia of the lower extremity is often done for cosmetic reasons, most such lesions produce symptoms ranging from numbness or paresthesia to pain (either aching or burning). The procedure is tedious and time-consuming, with a significant incidence of recurrence. However, because of the unattractive appearance of telangiectasia and the associated symptoms, there is a high patient demand for this form of therapy.

Our current cumulative experience includes a total of 85,639 injections in 1,842 patients between January 1982 and May 31, 1994. The average injection treatment consists of 10 injections at a single session. The majority of these patients had lower-extremity lesions, with a limited number in the face, chest wall, and breast. This chapter outlines our current management of these patients and describes our sclerotherapy technique.

PATIENT EVALUATION

Our current practice is to perform a complete preliminary history and physical, paying special attention to the arterial and venous system. The patient may have one or two noninvasive laboratory studies to complete the venous system assessment.

The patient is examined in the erect position (after 5-10 minutes of standing to allow for maximum inflation of bulging varicosities). Bulging varicosities and spider veins are accurately marked on leg diagrams during initial examination (Figs. 7-1 and 7-2). A copy of this diagram is on the chart during each injection treatment to facilitate an accurate record of injection locations.

The patient is then measured for custom-fitted support hose by the office staff. (In our clinic, this is performed by a specialized, pressure-gradient therapist.) A variety of brands are available. Over-the-counter types

are discouraged because the patient needs a stocking specific to his or her measurements. The patient brings the compression stocking to each injection appointment.

LABORATORY STUDIES

Initially, photoplethysmography (PPG) is used to evaluate venous valve function (and the degree of venous insufficiency). With proper technique, superficial

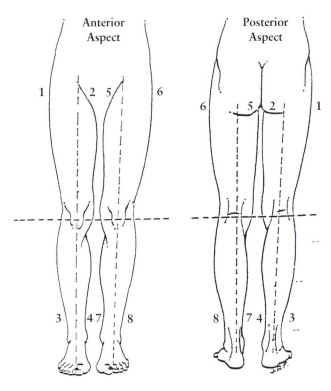

Fig. 7-1. Vein marking sheet, anterior and posterior aspects.

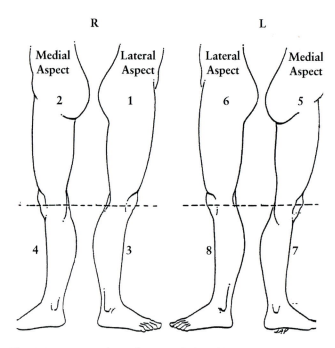

R   L

| Medial Aspect | Lateral Aspect | Lateral Aspect | Medial Aspect |

2   1   6   5

4   3   8   7

Fig. 7-2. Vein marking sheet, medial and lateral aspects.

and deep-venous insufficiency can be identified and managed prior to injection therapy. Doppler exam and duplex scan are used to determine points of reflux.

If there is any question of deep-vein thrombosis, we use the phleborheograph (PRG) as a screening study for recent venous occlusion. Positive PRG studies are then clarified by duplex scan. Duplex scanning is the best method for precisely assessing deep-venous occlusion, either acute or chronic, as well as locations of major venous reflux. The presence of chronic deep-vein occlusion is not a contraindication for sclerotherapy. However, the presence of acute, deep-vein thrombosis (DVT) is an absolute contraindication for sclerotherapy. If acute DVT is detected, sclerotherapy should be postponed for six months.

PATIENT PREPARATION

It is important to realize that although sclerotherapy is done for symptoms of pain, paresthesia, and so forth, the majority of patients have also come because of cosmetic concerns. Therefore, results are not based on the usual physician parameters of clinical improvement. Here, the patients' own assessment of results is important. In fact, the patients' decisions to proceed with treatment depends on their reaction to the degree of pain during the procedure and their assessment of the results. In sclerotherapy, patient comfort and patient satisfaction become critical factors in determining whether patients will continue with treatment. The physician's preinjection preparation of the patient becomes an important treatment component. A sup-

portive physician is important, but supportive and kind office personnel are equally important because they handle the many questions posed by these patients.

EXPLANATION OF RISK

Before injection sclerotherapy is performed, a comprehensive explanation of the procedure, with its attendant risks, is given to the patient (both verbal and written) at the time of preliminary examination (see Box 7-1.)

PRESCLEROTHERAPY PHOTOGRAPHY

Evaluation of results in sclerotherapy is highly subjective. Frequently, as the series of sclerotherapy treatments progresses, patients will forget how extensive their veins were prior to injection. Therefore, it is important to photograph all areas of planned injection prior to beginning sclerotherapy.

We use a Minolta-7000 35 mm camera with a macro 35-70 zoom lens. A data-back on the camera allows us to protect the patient's identity by assigning a code number to each patient. Prints are kept in the patient's file and are periodically reviewed with the patient. This photographic record also allows the treating physician to objectively evaluate improvement as treatment progresses.

SCLEROTHERAPY (OPERATIVE) PERMIT

A signed permit is obtained, even though this is an office procedure. Written permission to photograph the patient is also obtained. We use a single *Consent to Treatment* form that includes both injection and photography (see Box 7-2).

COMPRESSION STOCKINGS

Most spider telangiectasia are related to venous insufficiency with direct communication between telangiectatic channels and the deep-venous system. A leg that is not supported with a compression stocking following injection has a more rapid rate of recurrence of spider veins. Goldman and associates noted improvement in sclerotherapy results when compression was used. In our experience, the use of an adequate compression stocking has reduced recurrence by approximately 50%. Therefore, we maintain a full-time compression therapist on staff in our clinic, and we fit all

---

Box 7-1 Injection Therapy for Spider Veins

As you begin a program of sclerotherapy for your spider veins, we would like you to remember these things:

1. *Certain veins require 3 or 4 treatments before they disappear.*

   The principle of injection therapy for small skin veins is to inject a sclerosing (scarring) agent into the vein, which causes the vein wall to become inflamed and seal together. When the vein can no longer carry blood, it is no longer visible through the skin. Certain veins require 3 or 4 treatments before they disappear.

2. *There is occasional skin pigmentation (brown spots).*

   When the tiny needle is inserted into the vein for injection purposes, occasionally as the salt solution is injected, the vein will rupture, allowing this solution to leak into the surrounding tissue. This may result in a brown pigmented spot in the skin, which occasionally is permanent but usually disappears with time. It is usually small and no more obvious than the vein that was initially treated. However, you should be aware that this is a complication of injection of veins, although it only occurs in approximately 10% of the cases.

3. *There are rare occurrences of small skin ulcers that form after an injection.*

   Very rarely, an injection will be irritating enough to cause a small area of skin loss (or ulcer). In more than 70,000 injections, this complication has occurred 37 times. The size of a pencil eraser, these ulcers have healed without incident, leaving a small white scar.

4. *You will be required to support your legs after treatment.*

   After injection, your legs will be compressed with small gauze pads and a compression stocking (either calf high or pantyhose). This compression support stays in place for three days and two nights, during which time you will not be able to shower or have a complete bath. Then the stocking alone is used, while you resume daily showers, for an additional two weeks.

5. *Activities after injection.*

   During the injection treatments, your daily activities are not restricted. You may continue to work and perform your daily activities. However, aggressive exercising such as jogging, tennis, or high-impact aerobics should be avoided for one to three weeks following treatment.

6. *New spider veins may form, requiring subsequent treatment.*

   Because we function and work in the erect position, there is extra pressure on the veins of the leg. Thus, there is a tendency for new spider veins to form.

   Even after the majority of your veins have been removed by sclerotherapy, be aware that *new spider veins can develop.* We ask all our patients to return for periodic reevaluation so that any new veins can be injected before they become too large or too numerous.

7. *Flare formation.*

   Occasionally, immediately following injection, a new cluster of veins may form in close proximity to the vein just injected. This has the appearance of a "blush" in the skin. (These can usually be controlled by repeat injection).

---

patients for compression stockings at the time of preliminary evaluation. Patients are carefully instructed in application of pressure-gradient hose using rubber gloves, which prolongs the life of the hose.

If only below-knee injections are carried out, then 30-40 mmHg below-knee stockings can be used. If thigh injections are performed, a 20-30 mmHg pantyhose is fitted. If large, bulging veins are injected, 4- or 6-inch Ace bandages are snugly applied to the leg and the compression stocking is worn over the Ace bandage for the first three days.

The patient is required to wear the compression stocking for three days and two nights after treatment and is asked to avoid strenuous exercise. For the first three days, the injection sites are padded with gauze compression pads under the compression hose. After the first three days, the patient may take daily showers, but must wear the support stocking during the day for

two weeks, removing it only at night. When breast lesions are treated, they are compressed with elastic bandages overnight only.

On a long-term basis, we recommend that patients wear compression stockings for most of their standing activities. For women patients who are concerned about the appearance of compression stockings, several companies provide relatively sheer hose. Most patients are allowed to put aside the stockings in the hot summer months and for important social occasions. Our recommendation: "Wear them when you can hide them."

■ PATIENT SYMPTOMS

Weiss pointed out that most spider veins are symptomatic (numbness, paresthesia, aching and burning, pain, and so forth). Injection of veins almost always reduces or

---

Box 7-2   Consent to Treatment

I have been informed by the doctor of the nature of injection treatment of varicose veins. I understand the possible side effects, which include recurrence, skin pigmentation, skin ulcers, and localized clotted veins.

I authorize the doctor to take photographs of me before and after treatment and to permit such photographs to be used at the doctor's discretion for purposes of medical lecturing, research, or scientific publication, with the provision that I will not be identified.

FEES AND PAYMENT

Injections are billed individually at $_____ each.* Most treatments will not exceed twenty injections per appointment.

Due to the costs of providing this treatment, payment is expected at the time this service is rendered.

A deposit of $100.00 is required no later than (10) days prior to your scheduled appointment. This deposit confirms your appointment time and will be credited to your balance on your treatment day. All future scheduled appointments will also require a deposit in advance.

The balance at the time of treatment will then be that which exceeds the $100.00 deposit.

For your convenience, we do accept payment by cash, check, Visa, or Mastercard.

I understand all terms as written above, and I authorize the doctor to administer such treatment to me.

_____
PATIENT'S SIGNATURE

_____
DATE

*Due to the cost of providing these treatments, fees will be subject to change on an annual basis.

---

eliminates cutaneous symptoms, although the generalized aching of incompetent deep valves may persist.

▮ INDICATIONS FOR SCLEROTHERAPY

Vein Size

1. Small, bulging branch varicose veins, 3-6 mm.
2. Dilated venules (reticular veins), 1-3 mm.
3. Telangiectasia (spider veins), smaller than 1 mm.

Although controversial, many sclerotherapists do inject larger veins. We believe that larger varicose veins should be surgically excised using ¼-inch phlebectomy incisions. The results are very cosmetic, and the recur-

rence rate is lower with operation. Also, when injected, large veins often are complicated by skin pigmentation, which can be distressing to patients.

▮ CONTRAINDICATIONS TO SCLEROTHERAPY

The ongoing multicenter FDA trial on Sotradecol and Aethoxysklerol has established excellent exclusion criteria for the study. A partial list of these exclusion criteria serves as a reference for relative and absolute contraindications to injection.

Box 7-3   Preparation for Injection Treatment

1. On the day of your injections, bring your compression stockings.

2. Do not use bath oil or lotion on your legs the night before or the day of your injection treatment.

3. Dress in loose slacks, sweat pants, a dress, or skirt and comfortable loose shoes to accommodate the dressing.

4. If possible, bring loose fitting shorts to wear during the injection procedure.

5. Please call your insurance company if our office cannot advise you what your benefits are for this procedure.

Absolute Contraindications

1. Pregnancy.
2. Generalized systemic disease (cardiac, renal, hepatic, pulmonary, and collagen diseases and malignancies).
3. Advanced rheumatic disease, osteoarthritis, or any disease that interferes with patients' mobility.
4. Acute deep-vein thrombophlebitis.
5. Acute febrile illness.
6. Patients on anticoagulants.

Relative Contraindications

1. Patients with large varicose veins (larger than 6 mm in diameter). These are best treated with surgery, because they are often in communication with a source of venous reflux.
2. Elderly and sedentary patients (older than 80 years of age).
3. Arterial insufficiency of lower extremities (depending on location of planned injection).
4. Bronchial asthma or demonstrated allergies.
5. Obesity.
6. Acute superficial thrombophlebitis.

INSTRUCTIONS FOR SCLEROTHERAPY

Occasionally, patients are injected on the day of preliminary evaluation. However, the majority are scheduled for a separate sclerotherapy appointment on another day. Instructions on what to do to prepare for injection are given to the patients so they are adequately prepared for the injection procedure (see Box 7-3).

SCLEROSING SOLUTIONS

A variety of solutions is available for injection. Discussing the advantages of each as well as the drawbacks is beyond the scope of this chapter. Goldman's text on sclerotherapy is highly recommended for the interested reader. Hypertonic saline is recommended here because of the low risk of complications and generally excellent outcome.

INJECTION TECHNIQUE

1. The accuracy of intraluminal injection is enhanced by using 3-power loupes and a variable-intensity headlamp.

2. The patient lies flat in horizontal position on treatment table (either supine or prone, depending on location of venous lesion). A high-intensity light (preferably a headlamp) is used. Trendelenburg position and tourniquets are not necessary. The Ritter electric table is an excellent and relatively inexpensive table for injection.

3. The legs are photographed and recorded in a log book. Photos may be in a standing or horizontal position.

4. A copy of the initial venous mapping diagram is placed at the patient's bedside to allow accurate charting of all injections.

5. The leg area is prepped with aqueous Zephiran or similar colorless antiseptic solution. Infection after sclerotherapy is rare. One principal reason for prepping the site is to render the skin more transparent so the veins are more easily seen.

6. We use an injection solution of 23.4% saline (0.4 cc) plus 2% plain Xylocaine (0.1 cc) mixed in a 1 cc tuberculin syringe. (This solution is prepared in advance by injecting 2 cc of 2% plain Xylocaine into a 30 cc multiple dose vial of 23.4% saline. This dilutes the saline to 22%.)

7. Each injection is limited to 0.5 cc of solution to minimize the risk of injectant traversing the perforating vein and reaching the deep-venous system.

8. Retraction by assistant. Retracting the skin, to make it slightly taut, is helpful in assuring accurate injection (Fig. 7-3).

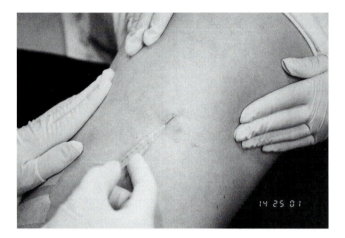

Fig. 7-3. Retraction of skin by an assistant facilitates needle entry into vein.

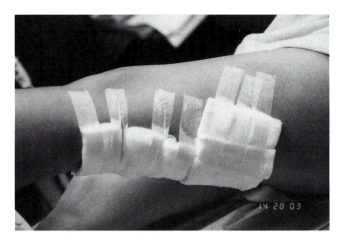

Fig. 7-4. Larger vein compression. Triple 4 × 4 gauze pad applied after injection.

9. A 30-gauge needle is used to enter the vein. A 3-power ocular loupe will facilitate accurate entry of the vein. *Injection must be intraluminal.* Perivenous injection can lead to pigmentation and skin necrosis. We bend the needle to 30 degrees to allow easier entry into the vein.

10. *The injection should be made slowly.* Watch the tip of the needle as you inject. The appearance of a small bubble suggesting extravasation means that individual injection should be terminated. If the physician watches carefully and stops immediately when extravasation occurs, these small bubbles subside without leaving a blemish. It is not necessary, and may be harmful, to dilute small extravasation bubbles.

11. Proper injection will result in blanching along the course of the injected vein. Erythema around the injected vein appears immediately after injection and indicates that the saline solution has been injected correctly throughout the distribution of the vein.

12. After injection, withdraw the needle and apply a pressure pad of three 4 × 4 gauze squares folded once. Use paper tape to hold the gauze pad in place.

13. Our sessions average 10 injections per treatment session and the usual patient has three sessions. We have injected as many as 80 sites in a single session if the patient has constraints of travel distance or time.

14. During the course of the sclerotherapy treatment, the injection sites are compressed with gauze pressure pads secured with paper tape. The compression hose are applied before the patient is allowed to get off the treatment table. Thus, the patient's legs are not permit-

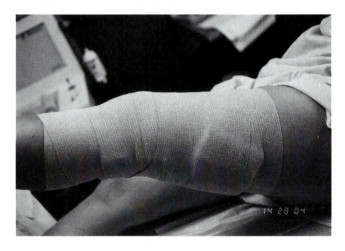

Fig. 7-5. Larger vein compression. Six-inch Ace bandage is wrapped over pads.

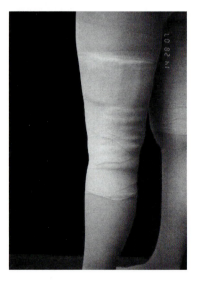

Fig. 7-6. Larger vein compression. Pressure-gradient hose applied over pads and 6-inch Ace bandage.

ted in the dependent position until the compression stocking is in place

The office nurse or compression therapist or a trained office assistant should put the stocking on the patients and instruct them in proper application and removal of the hose.

When larger veins are injected, we apply a 4- or 6-inch Ace bandage directly over the compression pads. The stocking is worn over this bandage for the first three days. This allows extra compression and reduces the likelihood of painful clot formation (Figs. 7-4 to 7-6).

Patients are then given a list of instructions to follow for the first two weeks after treatment (see Box 7-4).

■ POSTINJECTION COMPRESSION PADS

Figs. 7-7 and 7-8 illustrate injection of a popliteal reticular vein. We use a longitudinal pressure pad made of three 4 × 4 gauze squares. This is applied immediately after injection. The entire length of injected vein must be compressed, not just the point of needle entry. A 4 × 4 pad allows one to compress the entire length of vein to achieve more effective ablation (Fig. 7-9). If only a cotton ball is used at the needle-entry site, the remainder of the

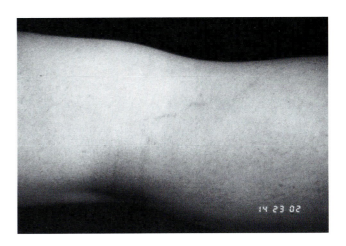

Fig. 7-7. Popliteal reticular vein.

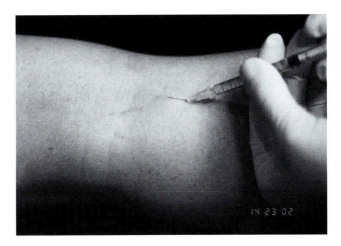

Fig. 7-8. Injection of popliteal reticular vein.

injected vein may refill, resulting in persistence of the injected vein and necessitating further injections (Fig. 7-10).

■ COMPLICATIONS OF SCLEROTHERAPY

1. Recurrence. Although it is not a complication of sclerotherapy, patients view recurrence as a complication. Remember, this is a gravity-related disorder and all varicose veins and spider veins tend to recur. If patients are warned prior to injection, they will be less concerned about recurrence and the need for repeat injections.
2. Pigmentation (3-5% of patients). This usually disappears in a few months, but may last as long as a year.
3. Telangiectatic matting or flare formation (1-3% of patients). These small venous blush

---

Box 7-4 Instructions to Follow After Injection Treatment

Days 1–3:

The stockings should remain in place for three days (including at night). The compression stocking is an important part of the treatment because it minimizes the blood reentering the injected vein. Elevate your legs as much as possible. Do not participate in jogging or high-impact aerobics at this time. At the end of the three days, you may remove the stocking and discard the gauze pads. (You may find standing in the shower a convenient way to loosen the tape holding the gauze pads to avoid blistering sensitive skin.) Do not be surprised if injected areas appear bruised at this time; that is normal with many skin types.

Days 4–14:

Continue to wear the compression stockings daily. Remove them at night to sleep. You may resume daily showers. Avoid jogging or high-impact aerobics during this time.

Days 15 on:

Continue to wear the compression stockings whenever you can because this will reduce the rate of recurrence of spider varicose veins.

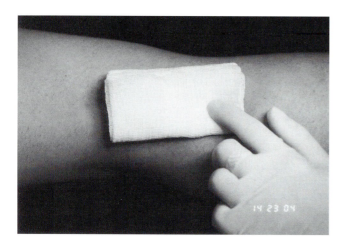

Fig. 7-9. This 4 × 4 pad compresses entire length of injected vein.

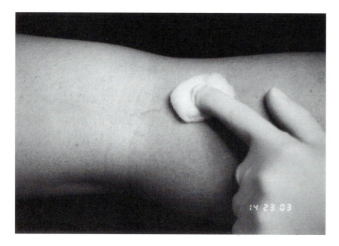

Fig. 7-10. Cotton ball compresses only needle-entry point and can result in persistence of distal noncompressed vein.

fomations near the injection site are very distressing to patients. The formations can effectively be eliminated by subsequent injection of dominant veins within the blush formation.

4. Ulceration 48/85,639 injections (1 per 1,784 injections). After hypertonic saline injection, these are usually small full-thickness ulcers less than 1 cm in diameter. They all heal in one to three months with minimal scarring. With some undiluted sclerosants, ulcers may be much larger.

5. Superficial phlebitis. Occasionally this is seen in veins adjacent to the injection site.

6. Deep-vein thrombosis. In our series, this has only occurred in two patients. Both were treated with anticoagulants and hospitalized and experienced no long-term sequelae. If the patient experiences unusual pain, fullness, or edema in the first few weeks after injection, noninvasive studies to rule out DVT should be carried out.

■ CONCLUSION

Our experience has suggested that injection sclerotherapy using hypertonic saline solution is a safe, relatively painless method of ablating small varicose veins, reticular venules, and spider telangiectasia, with minimal complications. The attending physician will have better results and happier patients if he or she remembers the following important concepts:

1. Although spider veins are symptomatic, most patients seek treatment because they are unhappy with the appearance of their legs. Be cautious and conservative so that you do not create a worse blemish than the patient already has.

2. Sclerotherapy should be viewed as a semicosmetic procedure and the patients' high expectations must be carefully considered.

3. Thoroughly discuss the risks with patients before the injections so they are fully aware of the protracted and tedious nature of sclerotherapy, as well as potential complications.

4. The effect of gravity and incompetent venous valves must always be remembered. Varicose veins and spider veins tend to recur. Wearing compression hose in the immediate postinjection period is mandatory. On a long-term basis, compression hose will significantly reduce recurrence.

5. Meticulous technique is essential in sclerotherapy.
   * Be sure your needle is in the vein.
   * Inject slowly.
   * Inject only 0.5 cc maximum per injection; avoid large bolus injection.
   * Watch the needle tip—stop injecting if there is extravasation.

With careful and precise techniques, most small spider veins and telangiectatic (spider) veins can be eliminated. Patient satisfaction with the procedure is high.

■ REFERENCES

1. Hobbs JT. The treatment of varicose veins: a random trial of injection compression therapy versus surgery. Br J Surg 55:777, 1968.

2. Pfeifer JR, Hawtof GD. Injection sclerotherapy and CO_2 laser sclerotherapy in the ablation of cutaneous spider veins of the lower extremity. Phlebology 4:231-240, 1989.

3. Faria JL, Morales IN. Histopathology of the telangiectasia associated with varicose veins. Dermatologica 127: 321-329, 1963.

4. Goldman MP, Beaudoing D, Marley W, Lopez L, Butie A. Compression in the treatment of leg telangiectasia: a preliminary report. J Dermatol Surg Oncol 16:4, 1990.

5. Fegan WG. Continuous compression technique of injecting varicose veins. Lancet 2:109, 1963.

6. Weiss RA, Weiss MA. Resolution of pain associated with varicose and telangiectatic leg veins after compression sclerotherapy. J Dermatol Surg Oncol 16:333-336, 1990.

7. Goldman P. Sclerotherapy. St Louis, 1991, Mosby Yearbook, Inc.

8. Williams RA, Wilson SE. Sclerosant treatment of varicose veins and deep vein thrombosis. Arch Surg 119: 1283-1285, 1984.

9. Browse NL, Burnard KG, Thomas ML,. Diseases of the veins, London 1988, Edward Arnold Publisher.

10. Bergan JT, Yao JST. Venous problems, Chicago, 1978, Year Book.

8

SCLEROTHERAPY FOR TELANGIECTASIAS

Neil Sadick

Small microvascular ectasias of the lower extremity usually measure 0.1 to 1 mm in diameter.[1] Class I telangiectasias appear as red linear vessels varying to dilated tortuous slightly elevated vessels often showing a reddish-bluish hue up to 1 mm in diameter. Class II venulectasias are slightly larger blue vessels measuring 1 to 2 mm in diameter. These small diameter vessels are often associated with Class III dilated subcutaneous reticular or Class III truncal varicosities. These are the major anatomic vessels that the present discussion of "microsclerotherapy techniques" will encompass[2] (Table 8-1).

The major goals of treating telangiectasia by means of sclerotherapy are (1) maximizing therapeutic efficacy, (2) minimizing the incidence of side effects, (3) minimizing patient discomfort, and (4) maximizing the number of treated veins per clinical session.

Table 8-1 Vessel Classification of Venous Disease

Type	Vessel Class	Diameter	Color
I	Telangiectasia "spider veins"	0.1–1 mm	Red
II	Venulectasia	1–2 mm	Violaceous, cyanotic
III	Reticular veins	2–4 mm	Cyanotic to blue
IV	Nonsaphenous varicose veins (usually related to incompetent perforators)	3–8 mm	Blue to blue-green
V	Saphenous varicose veins	7–8 mm	Blue to blue-green

■ PRESCLEROTHERAPY CONSULTATION

The best sclerotherapy patient is one who is an optimal candidate for achieving the most satisfactory therapeutic results as well as well educated. These goals may be best achieved by counseling the patient concerning (1) mechanical aspects of the procedure itself, (2) possible postsclerotherapy complications, (3) expected postsclerotherapy course and daily activity restrictions, and (4) realistic therapeutic expectations.

The pre-sclerotherapy consultation should include the following:

1. A careful, complete medical history including predisposing factors of varicose vein disease such as medications, genetic factors, elevated estrogen states, standing vocation, obesity, history of bleeding diatheses and thrombophlebitis, high-impact exercise, or other factors, that can affect the physician's treatment approach to the individual patient.[2] Elucidation of associated symptoms is also important and should be documented prior to sclerotherapy. A sample screening evaluation form is presented in Table 8-2.

2. A discussion of possible further diagnostic testing based upon physical examination to elucidate underlying saphenous or deep-venous disease including Doppler studies, photoplethysmography (PPG), light reflective rheography (LRR), or duplex ultrasound.

3. An explanation of mechanical aspects of the procedure.

4. A discussion of sclerosants that you expect to employ during sclerotherapy treatments, including a rationale and side effect profile of each chosen agent.

Table 8-2   Sclerotherapy Screening Evaluation

Symptoms of Telangiectatic/Varicose Veins

Aching pain	_____
Muscle fatigue	_____
Burning/itching	_____
Throbbing	_____
Night cramps	_____
Swelling	_____
Lower-extremity edema	_____
Lower-extremity swelling	_____
Lower-extremity discoloration	_____
Lower-extremity ulcers	_____
Lower-extremity phlebitis	_____
Cosmetic correction	_____

5. A description of possible side effects of the procedure. These should be divided into major versus minor complications as well as common versus infrequent anomalous treatment effects.

6. A discussion about the number of treatments and duration of treatment schedule so that realistic treatment expectations and activity schedule alterations can be implemented.

7. Postsclerotherapy compression and activity restriction explanations. This discussion should include the fact that sclerotherapy results are not noted immediately, and may not be seen for at least six to eight weeks after each treatment, and may require several treatments depending on the surface area of vascular ectasia involvement before significant improvement is clinically apparent.[4]

8. An explanation of estimated cost and insurance reimbursement considerations prior to beginning treatment.

9. A description of long-term prognosis and the treatment plan. This should include the long-term role of compression as well as minimizing predisposing factors discussed previously that might accelerate vesicular ectasia development in a genetically predisposed individual.

10. Obtainment of presclerotherapy photographic documentation.

11. Informed consent discussion and subsequent consent obtainment prior to beginning treatment.

■ MATERIALS: THE SCLEROTHERAPY SUITE (BOX 8-1)

The sclerotherapy suite should be a professional, well-equipped room that should maintain a sense of relaxation and assurance to the patient.

The following materials have been found to be extremely helpful in performing successful microsclerotherapy.[5,6]

1. *Power-operated table with stool.* Sclerotherapy of small veins is best accomplished when the patient is in the supine position. The easy up and down and lateral access motion of such a setup will ensure adequate physical access to difficult to reach microvascular locations and thus ensure improved clinical accuracy. Added benefits of such a set-up are that such table can be postured in the Trendelenberg or reverse Trendelenberg positions in the event a vasovagal reaction occurs and are helpful in mediating vascular dilitation (Fig. 8-1).

2. *Sclerotherapy tray,* set on a cart or Mayo-stand apparatus. The cart should be equipped with appropriately labeled sclerosants, needles, syringes, compression pads, and gauze pads (Fig. 8-2).

3. *Syringes.* Disposable 1 ml to 3 ml syringes (non leur-lock) are recommended (Becton-Dickinson & Co., Franklin Lakes, New Jersey). Insulin syringes ½ cc with 28-gauge ½-inch microfine needles, (Becton-Dickinson & Co., Rutherford, New Jersey) may be particularly helpful in treating areas of neoangiogenesis, "micromatting" where diminished injected pressures are preferable (Fig. 8-3).

Box 8-1   Materials for Performing Microsclerotherapy

Disposable 3 cc or tuberculin syringe
Fine needles (#30, #32, #33)
Sclerosant
Alcohol—½% acetic acid solution
Compression pads
Adhesive or elastic bandages
Support hose
Hyaluronidase
Magnifying source
Clear light source
Hand-held Doppler
Emergency resuscitation kit
Consent form
Anatomic region diagrammatic flow sheet

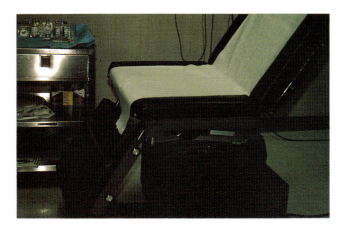

Fig. 8-1. Power-operated sclerotherapy table.

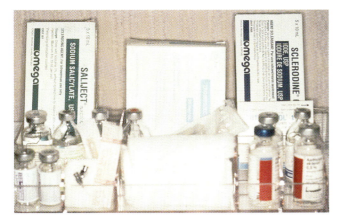

Fig. 8-2. Sclerotherapy tray equipped with labeled sclerosants, needles, compression pads, and sterile gauze.

4. *Needles.* The best and most durable needles for sclerotherapy are 30-gauge ½-inch hypodermic needles (Poly-Kote-metal bulb needle with silicone coated tri-beveled point [Acaderm Inc.; Ft. Lauderdale, Florida] or Air-Tite 30-gauge ½-inch needle [Air-Tite of Virginia, Inc.; Virginia Beach, VA]. Small gauge nondisposable autoclavable needles are available for treating areas of neoangiogenesis and Class I vessels 1-2 mm in diameter; however, these needles dull quickly and often bend easily so that it is difficult to achieve brisk cannulation of small vessels, which leads to frequent transection and thus adverse sequelae.

For improved results it is often helpful to change needles after every 10 to 15 injections particularly in areas of thickened rigid cutis (for example, inner thighs, popliteal fossa, feet, knees, or ankles) (Fig. 8-4).

5. Sclerosants should be correctly labeled to avert injection of an unwanted solution.

6. *Alcohol—½% acetic acid solution.* Application prior to treating vascular areas increases the index of refraction and thus improves visualization of vessels.[7]

7. *Magnifying source or spectacles.* Optivisor or Opticaid magnifiers or similar magnifiers with 2.5 power magnification may improve visualization and thus improve clinical results. A particularly helpful magnifying apparatus has been the diopter lamp (magnification of 5 diopters) (Dazor Manufacturing Corp, St. Louis, Missouri) (Fig. 8-5).

8. *Camera.* Several models are available that provide excellent results. Automatic cameras include the Yashica Medical Eye (Fig. 8-6). Other

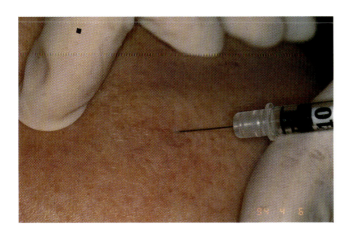

Fig. 8-3. Microfine insulin syringe (½ cc with 28-guage ½-inch microfine needle) used to treat microvascular and neoangiogenic micromatting vessels.

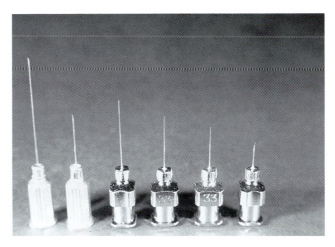

Fig. 8-4. Small gauge nondisposable autoclavable needles available for treating areas of neoangiogenesis and Class I–II vessels 1–2 mm in diameter.

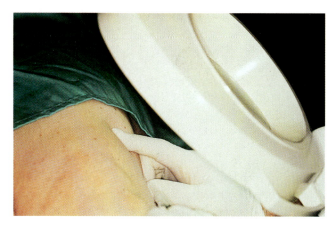

Fig. 8-5. Magnifying diopter lamp (5 diopters) can improve visualization of smaller vessels when performing microsclerotherapy.

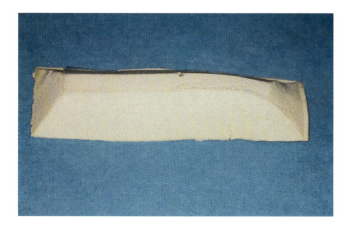

Fig. 8-7. STD-E pads can provide adequate postsclerotherapy compression when applied immediately after vessel cannulation.

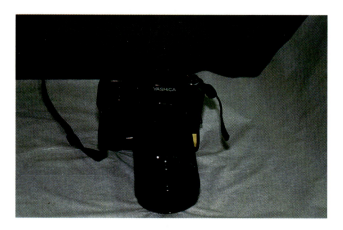

Fig. 8-6. Automatic macro lens Yashica Medical Eye camera produces excellent close-up photographic imaging for monitoring results of microsclerotherapy.

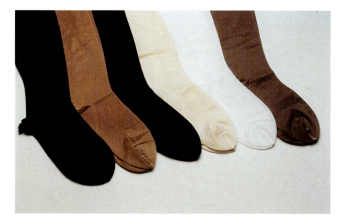

Fig. 8-8. Graduated compression stockings (15–40 mm Hg) should be continued for a minimum of 24 to 72 hours post sclerotherapy.

cameras that can be used in the manual focus mode include Autofocus Nikon 2020, 4004, 5005, 6006, and 8008 cameras equipped with Nikon speedlight 58-24 flashes.

9. *Clear light source.* Florescent lighting tends to provide shadow-free illumination. Overhead adjustable surgical spotlights are helpful in converging a concentrated light source on anatomic areas to be treated.

10. *Compression pads and tape.* Gauze pads 4 × 4 inch) STD-E pads (STD Pharmaceutical; Hereford, England), bandages, and cotton balls with micropore tape (5 mm ½-inch or Microfoam surgical tape [3M Medical-Surgical Division, St. Paul, MN] all may provide adequate postsclerotherapy compression (Fig. 8-7).

In flexural areas such as the popliteal fossae, using micropore tape beneath the Microfoam may minimize irritant and occlusive dermatitis.

11. *Graduated compressions stockings.* Post sclerotherapy compression of telangiectasias (15-40 mm Hg) should be continued for a minimum of 24 to 72 hours postsclerotherapy (preferably open toe) (Fig. 8-8).

This intervention has been shown to decrease postsclerotherapy hyperpigmentation by Goldman and associates.[8]

12. Informed consent form that includes all treatment risks, possible complications, and realistic treatment expectations.

13. Anatomic region diagrammatic flow charts (Fig. 8-9).

14. Normal saline, hyaluronic acid (150-300 IU), triamcinolone diacetonide, (40 mg/cc) and nitroglycerin paste. These should be available to treat suspected sites of extravasation.[9,10]

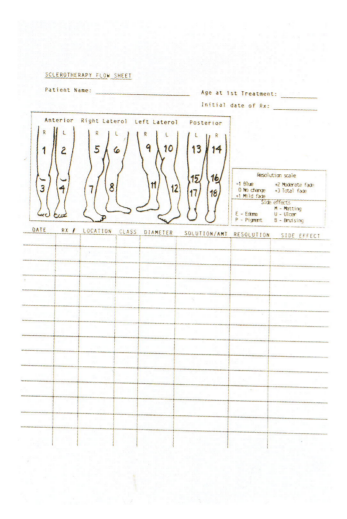

Fig. 8-9. Anatomic region diagrammatic flow chart used to monitor treatment sessions and clinical response to microsclerotherapy.

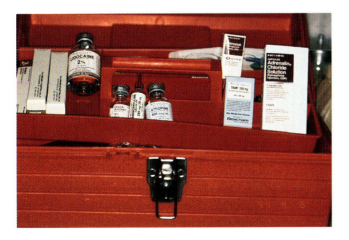

Fig. 8-10. Emergency cart equipped with colloid, analeptic and cardiotonic agents available to treat possible sclerotherapy emergencies such as anaphylaxis or arterial injection.

15. *Emergency Cart.* Such a vehicle should be equipped with Solumedrol, Ringer's lactate, normal saline, Benadryl, IV dextran, streptokinase, oral prazosin, hyaluronidase, nifedipine. Analeptic and cardiotonic agents should be available to treat possible anaphylaxis or inadvertent arterial injection (Fig. 8-10).

■ SEQUENCE OF EVENTS

Sclerotherapy should progress from treating the largest to the smallest vessels in an orderly, well-thought-out, systematic fashion (Box 8-2).[11]

In general, inject larger before smaller veins, that is injection of reticular veins feeding smaller nets of venules may eradicate these smaller vessels with less injections, thus minimizing the risks of side effects such as pigment dyschromia and ulceration. Similarly, areas of vascular arborization should be treated before single vessels are cannulated.

Box 8-2   Sclerotherapy of Varicose Veins—Sequence of Events

1. Physical examination.
2. Venous Doppler/light reflection rheography.
3. Consideration of duplex scanning or varicography if abnormal.
4. Elimination of high pressure inflow points:
   a. Saphenofemoral-popliteal junction
   b. Incompetent perforators
5. Sclerotherapy of large diameter varicose veins.
6. Sclerotherapy of communicating or reticular veins that feed "spider" telangiectasia.
7. Treatment of arborizing foci of venulectasia.
8. Sclerotherapy of "spider" telangiectasia.
9. Candela Pulse dye laser treatment of remaining fine telangiectasia and arteriolar telangiectasia.

Source: Modified from Goldman MP: Sclerotherapy treatment of varicose and telangiectatic leg veins, St Louis, 1991, Mosby-Year Book, Inc.

■ TREATMENT TECHNIQUES

Injection Quantities

The quantity of sclerosant injected produces an obliteration 1-6 cm from the point of injection.[12] More than 0.5 ml of sclerosant is never administered at a given injection site in order to avoid the risk of neo-angiogenesis (micromatting) occurring at a given anatomic site.[13]

Patient Positioning

Patients are usually positioned in a recumbent position or seated on a power-operated table with the sclerotherapist positioned at or below the level of the patient's knee. Inaccessible vessels on the lateral posterior thigh may be treated with the patient in the prone position (Fig. 8-11).

Injection Technique

A 30-gauge needle is employed initially, most commonly bent to an angle of 145° with the bevel positioned upward[14] (Fig. 8-12).

The skin is prepped either with alcohol or a combination of alcohol .5% acetic acid 1:1 to increase the index of refraction. Additional perfusion of the skin surface with sclerosant may also improve vascular visualization.[7]

Skin tension is an important factor in accurate and precise vessel cannulation. While the sclerotherapist holds the syringe in his or her dominant hand between the index and middle fingers, an assistant is often helpful to stretch the patient's skin in two opposing directions. The physician can achieve appropriate three-

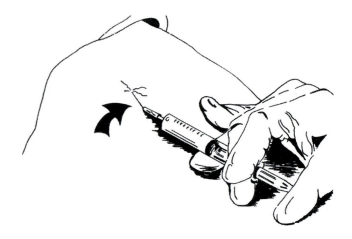

Fig. 8-12. Injection technique with 30-gauge needle bent 145° with the bevel positioned upward.

point tension alone when necessary by proper hand placement. The nondominant hand is used to stretch the skin adjacent to the treated vessel in two directions and then the fifth finger of the dominant hand exerts countertraction in a third direction (Fig. 8-13).

Brisk cannulation of veins causes minimal vascular trauma, less vasoconstriction, and less chance of extravasation of blood. Smaller veins can be made more pronounced at the surface by using an oversized, inflated, blood-pressure cuff.[2,4,14]

The following are several technique alternatives for treating telangiectasias:

1. *Aspiration technique.* Aspiration of a small amount of blood may ensure that the needle is truly in the vein. This can be recognized in the needle hub. Too strong aspiration can lead to vein collapse (Fig. 8-14, *A*).

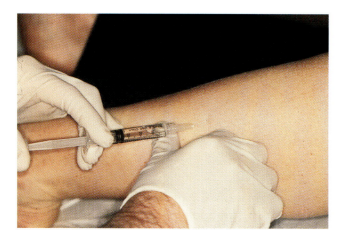

Fig. 8-11. Patient positioned in a recumbent position seated on a power-operated table.

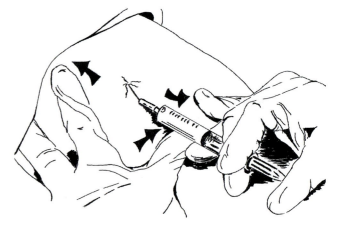

Fig. 8-13. Three-point tension technique with assistant present to stretch the patient's skin in two opposing directions, which ensures accurate and precise vessel cannulation.

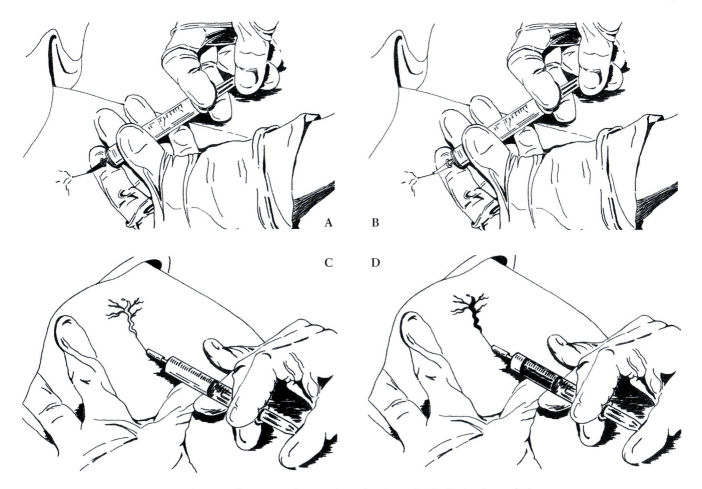

Fig. 8-14. Technique alternatives for treating telangiectasia. **A,** Aspiration technique: Aspiration of a small amount of blood ensures vessel cannulation. **B,** Puncture and feel technique: Feel of entering the vein by means of endothelial wall perforation is employed in this technique modification. **C,** Air bolus technique: Injection of 0.5 cc of air prior to introduction of sclerosant will show air in soft tissue if vessel cannulation has not been achieved. **D,** Empty vein technique: Emptying of treated vein decreases vascular volume and thus requires smaller volumes of sclerosant. The vein is emptied prior to vessel cannulation by kneading vessel with gentle pressure.

2. *Puncture and feel technique.* The feeling of having entered the vein by perforating the endothelial wall is another alternative technique modality. This technique is slightly more precarious for beginners; however, it can easily be mastered with time (Fig. 8-14, *B*).

3. *Air bolus technique.* Injection of 0.5 cc of air prior to introduction of sclerosant will show air in soft tissue rather than sclerosant (Fig. 8-14, *C*).

   However, too strong of a push may lead to luminal distention and damage.

4. *Empty vein technique* (Fig. 8-14, *D*). The persistence of telangiectasia and varicose veins after treatment is usually due to recanalization of the intramural thrombus that develops. This concept is more important when treating larger veins.

   Advantages of the technique are the following:

   a. An empty vein has minimal volume and therefore a smaller volume of sclerosant is necessary to contact the intraluminal surface compared with the volume needed for a distended vein.

b. Lower concentrations of sclerosant can be used since there is less blood in the vein to dilute the solution.

c. Lower injection pressures are required to deliver the solution into the vein.

5. *Sclerosant quantity.* Regardless of the technique employed, usually 2 cc of sclerosant is used in a 3 cc syringe. With continuous tissue tension applied the sclerosant is slowly injected. Since most telangiectasias are in the upper dermis a common problem in technique is to apply the needle too deep to the vessel or actually transect the vessel. If the vessel is appropriately cannulated, immediate blanching will occur in the treated vessel and its adjacent tributaries. If the needle is not within the vessel, extravasation will occur and either a superficial tissue wheal will occur or sclerosant will leak out onto the surface of the skin. Injection with the bevel of the needle up minimizes the chance of vascular transection by decreasing the vacuum produced by the bevel of the skin surface.

Slow injections and small volumes of sclerosant instilled at a given injection site regardless of sclerosant employed will minimize patient discomfort, extravasation, and damage to the deep-venous system.

6. *Choosing the optimal sclerosant.* In choosing the proper sclerosant for treating telangiectasia the physician must understand the relative strength of a sclerosant employed for a given vessel diameter, and should employ the minimal sclerosant concentration (MSC) for a given vessel diameter.[15,16]

Hypertonic saline 11.7% 23.4%, sodium tetradecyl sulfate (Sotradecol) 0.25-0.5%, and polidocanol (Aethoxysklerol) 0.25-0.5% are the most common sclerosing agents used in treating telangiectasia although the latter is not currently approved by the FDA. A summary of suggested sclerosing agents and recommended concentrations for various vessels diameter is presented in Table 8-3.

7. *Injection pressures.* Gentle injection of low volumes (less than 0.4 cc) of sclerosant that produce a small (less than 2 cm) blanch will improve sclerotherapy results while decreasing postsclerotherapy complications. This technique modification accomplishes this by decreasing vascular trauma and increasing the duration of contact between sclerosant and the vascular endothelium.[4] In general, it should take between 5 and 10 seconds to fill a given vessel. In addition, rapid pushes of large amounts of sclerosant can push the agent into deeper vessels, resulting in deep-venous thrombosis and possible pulmonary emboli. If the sclerosant appears to dissipate into the deeper venous system during the injection of superficial vessels, we should immediately stop the injection and begin cannulation at an adjacent site looking for superficial vessel blanching.

8. *Posttreatment modifications.* After sclerotherapy of telangiectasias, patients must recognize that burning, swelling, vein refilling, and urtication can occur that usually resolve rapidly.

After injection of hypertonic saline, cramping is particularly common and can be alleviated with gentle massage of the area, although most of this effect resolves spontaneously within 5 to 10 minutes.

Immediate postsclerotherapy urtication can be treated by a medium-potency, topical steroid such as flucinonide .05% or fluorandrelone .05% cream.

Areas of postsclerotherapy micromatting can occur particularly around the knees and

Table 8-3   Sclerosing Concentrations for Varicose and Telangiectatic Veins

Vein Diameter	Sclerosing Agent	Concentration
<0.4 mm	Polidocanol	0.25-0.5%
	Sodium tetradecyl sulfate	0.1-0.25%
	Hypertonic saline	10-15%
	Sodium morrhuate	1%
0.6–2 mm	Polidocanol	0.75-1%
	Sodium tetradecyl sulfate	0.25-0.5%
	Hypertonic saline	15-23.4%
	Sodium morrhuate	1%
3–5 mm	Polidocanol	1-2%
	Sodium tetradecyl sulfate	0.5-1%
	Sodium morrhuate	5%
>5 mm, perforators, saphenopopliteal and saphenofemoral junction	Polidocanol	3-5%
	Sodium tetradecyl sulfate	2-3%

Modified from: Goldman MP: Sclerotherapy treatment of varicose and telangiectatic leg veins, St. Louis, 1991, Mosby.

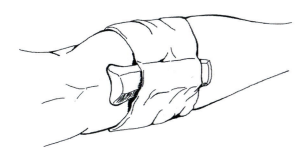

Fig. 8-15. Postsclerotherapy compression using STD-E pads applied over the injected vein and secured with a tape dressing.

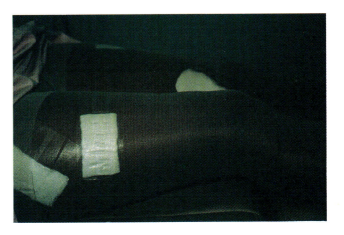

Fig. 8-16. Postsclerotherapy compression further carried out used 30–40 mm Hg graduated support hose for a minimum of 24 to 72 hours after each treatment session.

inner thighs. Although many of these vessels—up to 40%—will resolve spontaneously; if persistent they may be reinjected slowly under improved magnification using a 31- to 33-inch gauge nondisposable needle attached to a tuberculin syringe. More recently, good to excellent results have been documented int treating such microvessels using the Candela pulsed dye laser.[9]

9. *Posttreatment compression and guidelines.* Immediately following injection a cotton ball or foam-rubber compression pad (STD-E pad) is applied over the injected veins and secured with a tape dressing. (Fig. 8-15). This pad increases the relative pressure over the abnormal veins.[18]

Full compression following treatment of telangiectasia is then employed using a 30-40 mm Hg graduated stocking for a minimum of 24 to 72 hours after each treatment session.[19] (Fig. 8-16) Such compression has been shown to decrease postsclerotherapy pigmentation as well as theoretically serving to occlude the vascular lumina, decrease recanalization, and reduce the possibility of vascular thrombosis. More recently it has been suggested that compression can decrease the incidence of postsclerosis telangiectatic matting as well.[16,18] In general, following treatment of telangiectasia, patients can resume normal activity other than high-impact exercise for 48 hours. Walking, riding bicycles and low-impact aerobics are ideal exercise following sclerotherapy.

10. *Repeat treatment sessions.* A given anatomic area is not retreated for a period of 4 to 6 weeks to allow resolution of sclerotherapy-induced endosclerosis as well as allowing the physician to assess the clinical efficacy of a

given treatment using a given volume and concentration of a given sclerosing agent. Anatomic treatment charts documenting the anatomic region of veins treated at a given session, the size and number of vessels treated, and the amount of sclerosant employed at a given treatment session are extremely useful in this setting.

If telangiectasias are not responsive clinically to a given sclerosant at a given concentration one should either (1) look for areas of larger feeding such as reticular veins or perforators that might have initially been overlooked and treat these feeder sources first (Doppler guidance may be helpful in this clinical setting); (2) use a stronger concentration of the same sclerosing agent; or (3) choose a stronger sclerosing agent.[2,4,9,15]

■ COMPLICATION PROFILES IN SCLEROTHERAPY OF TELANGIECTASIA

Although it is beyond the scope of this review to detail the complications noted in small vessels compression sclerotherapy, a mention of the more important complications, their relative incidence, technique modifications that diminish their occurrence, and associated therapies are presented in Table 8-4.

■ CONCLUSION

Sclerotherapy of telangiectasias produces gratifying results when the appropriate patient is selected, appropriate sclerosant and appropriate sclerosant concentration (MSC) are used, and fastidious technique is employed.

Table 8-4 Microsclerotherapy Complications

A. Common Side Effects	Prevention/Treatment
1. Postsclerotherapy pigmentation	a. Use of minimal sclerosant concentration (MSC) for a given vessel diameter
	b. Fastidious technique
	c. Identification of patients with vascular fragility type syndromes such as Protein C, Protein S deficiency, antithrombin III deficiency, antiphospholipid antibody syndrome
	d. Use of low injection pressures
	e. Postsclerotherapy compression
	f. Recognition, incision, and drainage of postsclerotherapy thrombi within 48 hours
	g. Candela pigmented dye laser [20]
	h. Copper vapor laser[21]
2. Lower-extremity edema	a. Limiting the quantity of sclerosing solution to 1 cc per ankle
	b. Use of post sclerotherapy 30–40 mm Hg graduated compression
3. Telangiectatic matting	a. Limiting hyperestrogen states (such as pregnancy, oral contraceptives)
	b. Observation because as many as ⅓ of vessels resolve with a year
	c. Treatment with low concentrations of sclerosant employing a 31"-33" gauge needle
	d. Treatment with the Candela pulsed dye laser
4. Localized urticaria	a. Pretreatment with H1 antihistamines
	b. Medium potency topical corticosteroids
5. Hirsutism	
6. Vasovagal reactions	a. Eating a light meal prior to each treatment session
	b. Presclerotherapy monitoring of blood pressure and heart rate
	c. Documentation of vasovagal tendencies
	d. Adequate ventilation
	e. Consideration of treatment with patient in a totally supine position
	f. Careful physician and patient communication
7. Patient discomfort	a. More common with 23.4% hypertonic saline and may be diminished by using 11.7% HS for treatment of vessels <4 mm in diameter
	b. Kneading of painful areas by nursing personnel immediately post injection

B. Uncommon Side Effects	Prevention/Treatment
1. Ulceration	a. Fastidious technique
	b. Installation of 150–300 U of Hyaluronidase immediately to surrounding area if extravasation is suspected
	c. Topical nitroglycerin
	d. Domeboro's solution 5%/Bactroban ointment
	e. Hydrocolloid dressings (Duoderm, Allervyne)
	f. Early primary excision of ulcers
2. Systemic hypersensitivity	a. Having patient sit in waiting room for 15–30 minutes following treatment sessions when using agents other than hypertonic saline
	b. An adequate treatment cart available (epinephrine, Benadryl, oxygen, Medrol, saline, Ringer's lactate)
3. Thrombophlebitis	a. Adequate post sclerotherapy compression
	b. Evaluation of postsclerotherapy thrombi
	c. Tepid compresses
	d. Nonsteroidal antiinflammatory agents
4. Arterial injection with secondary necrosis	a. Proper visulation of blood in the needle bevel
	b. Treatment that includes immediate heparinization and support pressures
	c. IV dextran
	d. IV streptokinase
	e. Oral prazosin
	f. Hydralazine
	g. Nifedipine
5. Problems related to bandaging such as ulcers, contact dermatitis, pressure blisters	a. Checking tightness of bandages only if patients complain of increasing pain
	b. Use of beveled rubber foam pads
6. Pulmonary emboli	a. Rare in small vessel sclerotherapy
	b. Injection of small amounts of sclerosant agent
	c. Adequate compression
	d. Postsclerotherapy ambulation
7. Nerve damage	a. Watching for the saphenous and sural nerves
	b. Nonsteroidal antiinflammatory agents

■ REFERENCES

1. Goldman MP: Treatment of telangiectasia: a review, J Am Acad Dermatol 17:167-182, 1987.

2. Goldman MP: Sclerotherapy treatment for varicose and telangiectatic leg veins. In Coleman MP, Havile CW, Pit TN, Asken S, Becker BC, editors: Cosmetic surgery of the skin: principles and techniques. Philadelphia, 1990.

3. Sadick NS: Predisposing factors of varicose and telangiectatic leg veins, J Dermatol Surg Oncol 18:883-886, 1992.

4. Goldman MP: Clinical methods for sclerotherapy of telangiectasias. In Goldman, MP et al.: Sclerotherapy: treatment of varicose and telangiectatic leg veins, p. 307-324. St Louis, 1991, Mosby–Year Book.

5. Duffy DM: Setting-up a vein treatment center: incorporating sclerotherapy into the dermatologic practice, Sem Dermatol 12:150-158, 1993.

6. Guex JJ: Microsclerotherapy, Sem Dermatol 12:129-134, 1992.

7. Scarborough DA, Bisaccia E: Sclerotherapy-translucidation of the skin prior to injection, J Dermatol Surg Oncol 15:498-499, 1989.

8. Bodin EL: Sclerotherapy, Sem Dermatol 6:238-248, 1987.

9. Goldman MP: Adverse sequelae of sclerotherapy treatment of varicose and telangiectatic leg veins. In Bergan JJ, Goldman MP, editors: Varicose veins and telangiectatic diagnosis and treatment, p. 259-290. St Louis, 1993, Quality Medical Publishing.

10. Zimmet SE: The prevention of cutaneous necrosis following extravasation of hypertonic saline and sodium tetradecyl sulfate, J Dermatol Surg Oncol 19:641-646, 1993.

11. Goldman MP: Advances in sclerotherapy: treatment of varicose and telangiectatic leg veins, Am J Cosmetic Surg 9:238-241, 1992.

12. Sadick NS. Hyperosmolar versus detergent sclerosing agents in sclerotherapy: Effect on distal vessel obliteration, J Dermatol Surg Oncol 20:1-4, 1994.

13. Duffy DM: Small vessel sclerotherapy: an overview, Advan Dermatol 3:221-242, 1988.

14. Bodian EL: Techniques of sclerotherapy for sunburst venous blemishes, J Dermatol Surg Oncol 11:696-704, 1985.

15. Sadick NS: Sclerotherapy of varicose and telangiectatic leg veins: minimal sclerosant concentration of hypertonic saline and its relationship to vessel diameter, J Dermatol Surg Oncol 17:65-70, 1991.

16. Duffy DM: Sclerotherapy, J Clin Dermatol 10:373-380, 1992.

17. Goldman MP, Fitzpatrick RE: Pulsed dye laser treatment of leg telangiectasia with and without simultaneous sclerotherapy, J Dermatol Surg Oncol 16:338-344, 1990.

18. Goldman MP, Beaudoing D, Marley W, Lopez IL, Butie A: Compression in the treatment of leg telangiectasia: a preliminary report, J Dermatol Surg Oncol 16:322-325, 1990.

19. Stanley PR, Bickerton DR, Campbell WB: Injection sclerotherapy for varicose veins: a comparison of materials for applying local compression, Phlebol 6:37-39, 1990.

20. Goldman MP: Post sclerotherapy hyperpigmentation: treatment with a flash-lamp excited pulsed dye laser, J Dermatol Surg Oncol 18:417-422, 1992.

21. Thibault P, Wlodarczuyk J: Post sclerotherapy hyperpigmentation: the role of serum ferritin levels and the effectiveness of treatment with the copper vapor laser, J Dermatol Surg Oncol 18:47-52, 1992.

9

SCLEROTHERAPY OF TELANGIECTASIAS: ITALIAN AND EUROPEAN TECHNIQUES

Mihael Georgiev

Leg telangiectasias appear in different patterns as indicated in Chapter 1. They can develop from larger vein incompetence and can be connected to incompetent superficial or perforating veins. In such cases, the telangiectasias are often arranged in dense networks (webs or flares). Selective compression of the feeder vein, similar to the Trendelenburg test for large varicose veins or the venous Doppler examination, can prove that the flare is fed by that particular vein in many cases (Fig. 9-1, A, B). In such instances, avulsion or sclerosis of the feeder vein invariably reduces the number and size of the dependent telangiectasias (Fig. 9-2, A, B). In addition, large, blue venulectasias can be hooked and avulsed. Subepidermal "scratching" of the telangiectatic flare with a No. 1 Muller hook during phlebectomy can cause further mechanical destruction of venules (Fig. 9-3). However, while these procedures greatly enhance the elimination of telangiectasias, they rarely clear the skin completely. Thus, different methods must be employed after phlebectomy to achieve the best cosmetic result.

EFFECTS OF SCLEROSING INJECTION

The effects of a sclerosing injection on venules and perivenular tissues may vary considerably between patients and even between different sites on the same patient. This is due to different vessel and tissue sensitivity (fragility) to the action of the sclerosant.[1]

It is not uncommon for telangiectasias to disappear completely after a single injection, provided that the vessel wall has been sufficiently damaged and the venule has collapsed and been kept empty by adequate postinjection compression. This is, of course, the best possible outcome (Fig. 9-4). In many cases, however, endothelial damage is followed by blood clotting in the venule. The

resulting coagulum is easily seen, especially in large telangiectasias, and it may appear green, blue, or black. If the venule is still visible a few days after injection, vessel damage and thrombus formation are confirmed by failure to empty the venule by digital pressure.

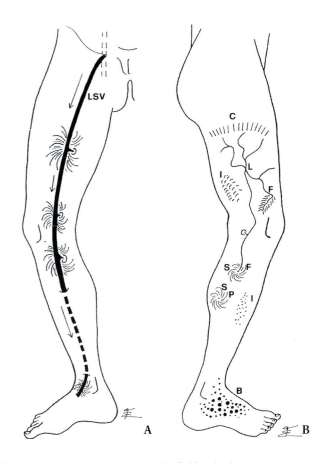

Fig. 9-1. A, telangiectasia may be fed by the long-greater saphenous vein or **B,** reticular veins.

79

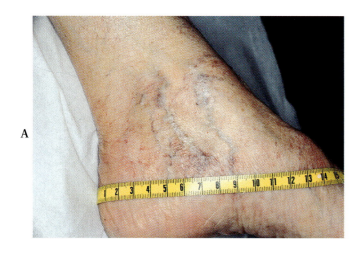

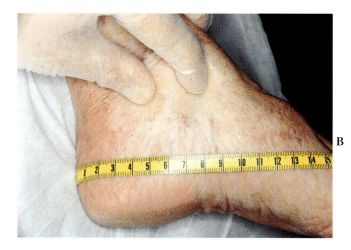

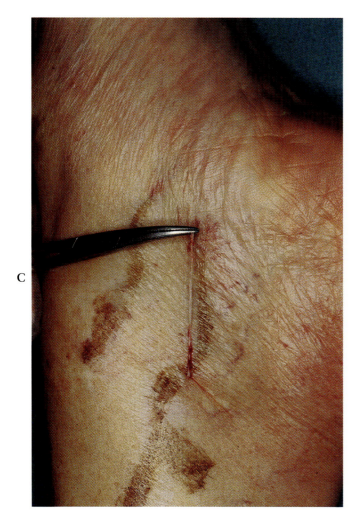

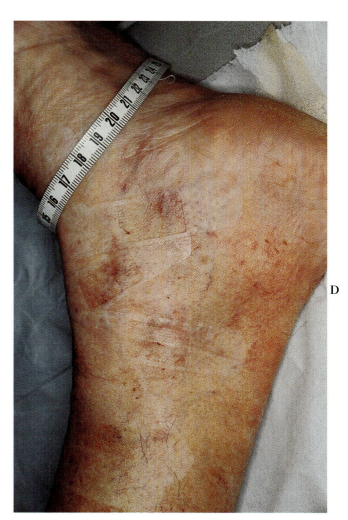

Fig. 9-2. Phlebectomy for treatment of telangiectasias filled by an incompetent dermal (reticular) vein. **A,** Ankle telangiectatic flare (tiny, bright red telangiectasias). **B,** Remain empty after digital compression of the feeder veins. **C,** Avulsion of the feeder vein by needle puncture phlebectomy. **D,** Reduced number and size of dependent telangiectasias shown 5 days after phlebectomy.

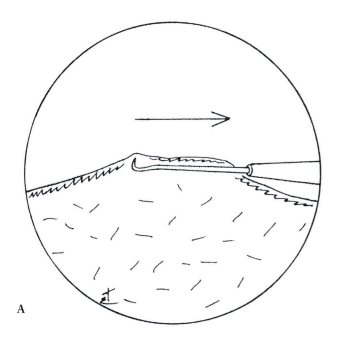

A

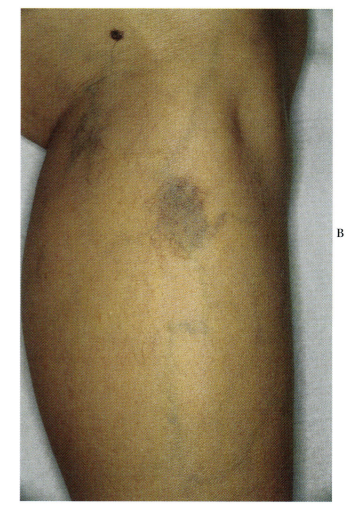

B

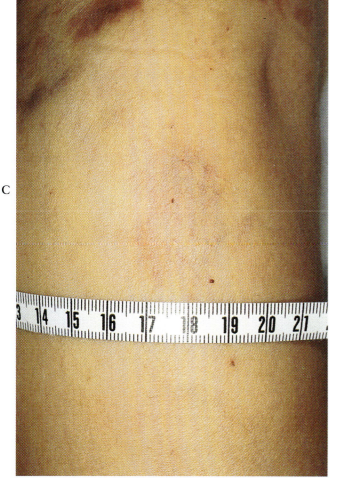

C

Fig. 9-3. Phlebectomy for treatment of leg telangiectasias. **A,** In addition to feeder (reticular) vein avulsion, large telangiectasias can be "scraped" with a No. 1 Muller phlebectomy hook as shown here. **B,** Telangiectatic flare crossed by an incompetent dermal (reticular) vein. **C,** Five days after avulsion of the reticular vein and scratching of the telangiectatic flare with a No. 1 Muller hook. Some bruising in the upper left angle of photograph. Signs of needle punctures (phlebectomy incisions) are still visible. Telangiectasias are greatly reduced in number and size but need further sclerotherapy to completely disappear. (From: Ricci S, Georgiev M, editors: Ambulatory phlebectomy: a practical guide for treating varicose veins. St Louis, 1994, Mosby.)

Vessel damage with thrombus formation is a favorable response that leads to the vessel's destruction. However, this often causes perivenular skin inflammation, and it can take a few weeks or even months for the thrombosed telangiectasia and signs of skin inflammation to disappear (Fig. 9-5). In other cases, there is some venular fading after each treatment without

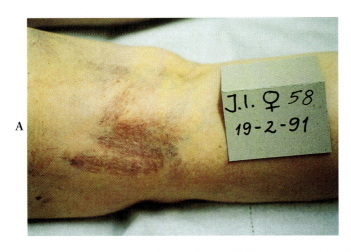
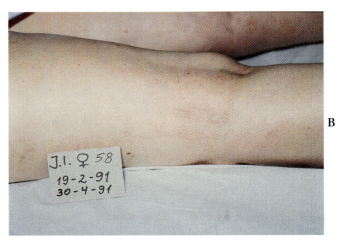

Fig. 9-4. Massive rapid destruction of telangiectasias. **A,** Dense telangiectatic flare.
B, Complete disappearance of telangiectasias four weeks later after three sessions with 0.5%
polidocanol, local compression padding, and Class III compression stocking worn during the
daytime. Note the absence of visible inflammatory reaction.

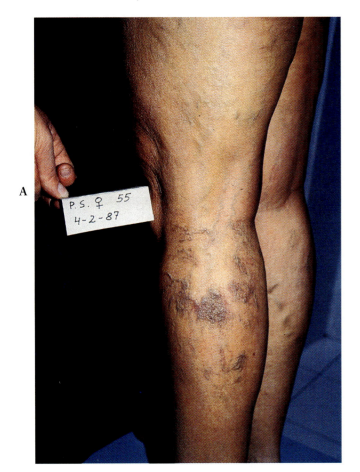
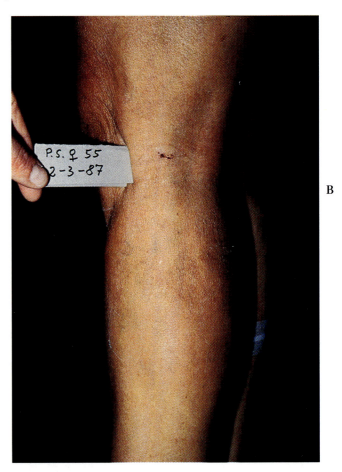

Fig. 9-5. Post injection thrombosis. **A,** Seven days after injection with chromated glycerin.
Venule damage with thrombus formation, bruising, and perivenular inflammatory reaction.
Note undamaged telangiectasia close to the damaged ones. This demonstrates the importance
of injecting extremely small amounts (0.01–0.2 ml) of sclerosant per injection. An attempt to
inject a larger amount to damage a larger area of telangiectasias might cause excessive inflammation or irreversible skin damage at the site of injection. **B,** Four weeks after evacuation of
coagula by 26-gauge needle puncture and continuous daytime compression with a Class III
stocking. Red/brown pigmentation is still present (early post sclerotherapy hyperpigmentation), but faded away completely three months later.

demonstrable obliteration or thrombosis. Venules tend to fade gradually after repeated injections. Sometimes, however, telangiectasias appear unchanged after injection. This implies that the type, concentration, and amount of sclerosing solution was not been sufficient to cause vessel wall damage. In this case, a more concentrated or stronger sclerosing solution is needed.

◼ SCLEROSING SOLUTIONS

We employ two sclerosing solutions: 72% glycerin and polidocanol.

Glycerin for sclerosing injections was commercially available until recently under the name Scleremo (SCL) as 5 ml vials containing 72% glycerin, chromated with chrome allume at 1.11%. SCL has been employed in Europe for decades, but is no longer available. Pure sterile glycerin at 72% can be successfully employed instead of chromated glycerin[2] and is commercially available in 3 ml vials from Amodont s.a.s., Sesto Fiorintino, Firenze, Italy, but not in the United States.

Polidocanol (POL, dihydroxypolyethoxydodecane, Aethoxysklerol, Kreussler, Germany) is employed at 0.5%. It is commercially available in various size vials and concentrations. The more concentrated solution (1%) is only rarely injected into telangiectasias.

◼ SYRINGES

Though modern disposable syringes have smooth-moving, low-resistance plungers, I prefer all-glass syringes, which offer less resistance to piston advancement. This allows better feel during injection. The only disadvantage of glass syringes is that they have to be cleaned and sterilized between patients. For this reason, we keep them first for a few hours in a disinfectant solution (5% sodium hypochlorite is adequate). They are then rinsed, dried, and wrapped individually in aluminum foil and sterilized in a dry heat device.

One to 3 ml syringes may be employed. I prefer 1 ml insulin-type syringes because they permit better positioning of the needle almost parallel to the skin without requiring the needle to be bent. This affords better control of the injected quantity, making it easy to inject amounts less than 0.1 ml.

◼ HYPODERMIC NEEDLES

We employ 26-gauge (26 G ½, 0.45 × 12 mm, Terumo Corporation, Japan) and 30-gauge (Mesoram 30 GT ½, 0.30 × 13 mm, RAM, Mirandola, Modena, Italy) disposable needles.

◼ COMPRESSION MATERIAL

Compression includes adhesive elastic bandages, short-stretch compression bandages, Class I (18-21 mm) elastic stockings, Class II (36-46 mm) compression stockings, and normal nylon stockings.

◼ CHOICE OF SCLEROSANT

Chromated glycerin has been shown experimentally and clinically to be milder than 0.5% polidocanol.[2-4] We now employ 72% glycerin instead of chromated glycerin and obtain the same clinical results. It will practically never cause skin necrosis. Skin inflammation is also absent or mild. Postsclerotherapy hyperpigmentation is infrequent and almost invariably fades with time. Prior to injecting 72% glycerin, we add 0.3 ml of 2% mepivacaine and epinephrine 1:100,00 to the 3 ml vial of glycerin to minimize pain and cramping that may follow glycerin injection. This 10% dilution also lowers the density of the solution and makes it easier to inject, especially if disposable (plastic) syringes and 30-gauge needles are used.

It is possible to employ only glycerin with its advantage of minimizing the risks of skin necrosis, inflammation, and hyperpigmentation. However, more treatment sessions are often necessary and in some cases, a stronger sclerosing agent (that is, polidocanol) is needed to achieve the desired result.

Polidocanol (Aethoxysklerol, POL) is employed at 0.5%. Higher concentrations (0.75% or 1%) are rarely injected into telangiectasias. Though intradermal injection of 0.5 to 1.0% polidocanol is usually well tolerated, occasionally even the 0.5% solution causes a strong inflammatory reaction or skin ulceration. When both sclerosing agents are employed, the choice of which one to inject is made as follows:

The first treatment for a patient in whom the reason for a sclero-inflammatory reaction is unknown is considered a "trial session." Glycerin (the milder sclerosant) is injected to test for vessel fragility and intensity of the accompanying inflammatory reaction. Two to seven days later, the patient is seen again, the reaction to the "test" injection observed, and the treatment continued with either glycerin or the stronger POL, depending on the response. If all (or most) of the injected venules are damaged and there is a strong inflammatory reaction (perivenous edema, hyperemia, brown staining), changing the glycerin to a stronger sclerosant is unwise, and treatment is continued with glycerin.

Approximately 30% of our patients have strong inflammatory reactions and are treated solely with glycerin. A stronger sclerosant (POL) may increase the incidence of postsclerotherapy hyperpigmentation.[2]

If, on the contrary, the effect of glycerin is absent or mild (only a few vessels damaged) or there is no inflammatory skin reaction, SCL is replaced with the stronger POL. We treat more than 70% of our patients with POL. POL is, therefore, our main sclerosing agent, glycerin being employed only to "select" the patients who react with massive destruction of venules and strong perivenular inflammatory reaction. Extending the use of glycerin beyond these "hypersensitive" patients prolongs treatment (more sessions) without reducing postsclerotherapy hyperpigmentation.[2]

PATIENT POSITION AND SKIN PREPARATION

The patient is positioned flat with the area to inject brought as closely as possible to horizontal. In cases of very large, dense, and widespread telangiectasias especially on the lower leg and foot, we inject the foot elevated to reduce venous pooling and blood clotting. This enhances the action of the sclerosant agent on the vessel wall. The patient must be instructed to keep the skin free of body lotion or other creams, or the tapes will not stay in place. Prior to injection, the skin is wiped with alcohol and then dried. This makes the skin more transparent and permits better visualization of telangiectasias.

INJECTION TECHNIQUE

The advantage of a 26-gauge needle is that the bevel is visible to the naked eye so that correct intravenous position can be checked without magnification. Direct observation of the bevel in the telangiectasia is possible because the latter is so superficial that the epidermal layer covering it is "transparent." We employ Terumo 26 G ½″ (0.45 × 12 mm) disposable needles (longer needles are more difficult to point) and then perform injection as follows:

For the right-handed operator, the skin is pulled tight by an assistant or the operator's left hand to avoid skin deformation with distortion of the venule upon pressure of the needle tip. Obviously, the skin must not be stretched so much that it completely flattens the venule and makes it invisible. The syringe is held at the base between the index and third fingers with the hand in the semiprone position, firmly supported against the skin to avoid tremor and uncontrolled movement. The distal part of the syringe and the needle are also supported against the skin.

Puncture is performed by merely advancing the syringe on the skin until only the bevel enters into the telangiectasia (about 2 mm). When the needle tip is correctly positioned, its opening is clearly seen as a "dark window" under the thinned epidermis covering the telangiectasia. No attempt is made to introduce the needle further into the skin and aspiration is not performed since these maneuvers often break the venule. If a glass syringe is used, spontaneous backflow of blood into the syringe might occur due to minimal resistance to piston movement. At this point, the injection is started by slight pressure on the piston with the thumb. No resistance to injection, immediate clearance of the injected venules (as blood is replaced by sclerosant), and no (or very little) pain confirms that correct intravenous injection is being performed.

On the other hand, resistance to injection, an appearance of a small, raised wheal at the needle tip, or unusual pain reported by the patient indicate perivenous injection. In this case, it is better to stop injecting immediately and withdraw the needle. This may also be done by keeping the piston under slight pressure while slowly withdrawing the needle. If the venule has been transfixed during needle penetration, it might still be injected during this slow withdrawal motion. However, if proper injection is not achieved, it is better to stop injecting and try again rather than inject with an uncertain needle position.

Injecting a small amount of air before the sclerosant can help confirm correct needle position. If no bubbles are seen in the venule, injection is stopped.

When injection is completed and the needle withdrawn, a cottonball is applied over the treated area, pressed firmly, and secured with one-inch paper tape stretched with slight tension over the cottonball. An assistant can keep a few cottonballs pressed again the skin to assist taping. We find it advantageous to maintain digital pressure for a few minutes over dense networks of venules. The patient is instructed to remove the cottonballs after 24 hours unless there is redness, pain, or blister formation around the tapes in which case the cottonballs are immediately removed.

Confirmation of intravenous position of the 26-gauge needle permits many injections in a short time. With some experience, even telangiectasias with diameters smaller than that of the needle can be injected. However, when vessel cannulation with a 26-gauge needle repeatedly fails (because telangiectasias are too small), successful injections may be performed with a 30-gauge needle.

The intravenous position of the 30-gauge needle is difficult to confirm without magnification. However, correct needle position is possible without magnification. After advancing the needle approximately 1-2 mm, gently press against the piston. If the needle is correctly placed, the telangiectasia immediately clears and no wheal is raised. Gentle to and fro motion of the needle, while pressing against the piston, may assist intraluminal injection. We use the 30-gauge needle to inject the smallest, bright-red telangiectasias, especially those left after destruction of the larger ones. Injection of larger telangiectasias with 30-gauge needles does not appear to be advantageous and is even more difficult than with the 26-gauge needle. Both 26- and 30-gauge needles may become dull after repeated injections. Therefore, we recommend changing the needle often.

INJECTION OF RETICULAR VEINS

The possibility of avulsion of reticular (1-3 mm) dermal veins through needle punctures with virtually no visible scars greatly reduces the need to treat them by sclerotherapy. However, occasionally it may be necessary to inject into reticular veins such as for "borderline" venules for which sclerotherapy can just be efficacious or for small reticular veins left after phlebectomy of the larger ones. Reticular veins are injected by a method similar to common intravenous injection. Intravenous position of the needle is confirmed by aspiration of blood and by injection of a small amount of air before the sclerosant. As with telangiectasias, chromated glycerin is injected first and then, in the case of failure, 1% polidocanol is used.

AMOUNT OF SCLEROSANT

There is no rule regarding the amount of sclerosant per injection. Injection is stopped when telangiectasias in an area of approximately 2.0 to 2.5 cm diameter have been "cleared." This is usually achieved with 0.5 to 0.2 ml per injection. Such quantity can clear long linear telangiectasias as far as 10 cm away from the injection point.

Injecting small amounts of sclerosing solution is the best way to keep the intensity and extension of the sclerosing agent effect under control. This helps avoid phlebitis and thrombosis far from the injection sites and in veins not targeted for treatment. With such small amounts per injection the number of injections one can perform is practically unlimited. Except for the first session when some caution is advisable, we usually inject all telangiectasias. Sometimes this is more than 50 injections per session. Larger amounts of sclerosant (as much as 0.5 ml) can be injected into dense networks (flares) of large telangiectasias, especially if the patient is known to have a mild reaction or when previous injections have proven inefficacious.

POSTINJECTION COMPRESSION

The goal of postinjection compression is to minimize skin inflammation and its sequelae, telangiectatic matting, and hyperpigmentation. Compression also helps maintain an empty venule. The importance of adequate postinjection compression cannot be over-emphasized. The only problem with compression is that patients are usually not enthusiastic about it.

The need and importance of compression varies according to the type of venules and individual response to sclerosing injections. Patients with no (or minimal) inflammatory reaction can be treated with minimal or short-lasting compression, whereas those with strong inflammatory reactions may need stronger and longer-lasting compression. In many cases, adequate compression is indispensable for achieving an acceptable result. We see many patients who were treated previously without success (and without compression). However, even in cases with the most favorable course of treatment, compression is still useful. It permits more intensive treatment and more predictable results. As Sigg said, "good results of sclerotherapy are the results of good compression."[5] For these reasons, we apply compression to all treated patients.

The exact method of compression may vary and depends much on the preference of the operator. Comparable results may be obtained by different compression methods. Guidelines for our decisions regarding the type and duration of postinjection compression are as follows:

Full-Length Compression

When telangiectasias are spread over the entire limb, full-length compression is used. This may be achieved by Class III (36-46 mm) single-leg stockings or Class I (18-21 mm) pantyhose. If a Class III stocking is used, a normal nylon stocking is applied first and then the compression stocking is applied over it. With this technique, the latter slides easily over the nylon stocking without removing the cottonballs taped over the injection sites.

The compression stocking is worn during the daytime. The patient puts it on in the morning and takes it off in the evening. Some practice is needed to properly apply and remove Class III compression stockings, and the patient must be adequately instructed in the office.

With very widespread telangiectasias, many injections in a single session, or signs of skin inflammation, the patient is advised to sleep for one or two nights after injection with a Class I compression stocking. If there is no visible skin inflammation, the patient may be allowed to wear a Class III stocking for the first two to three days and then replace it with a Class I pantyhose for the rest of the week.

An alternative compression method is to apply local compression pads over the injected sites and secure these with strips of adhesive bandage for three to seven days. The patient then applies Class I pantyhose over this and continues to wear it after the removal of the compression pads until the end of the treatment. In many cases, such a regime achieves adequate compression over the injected venules without the need for stronger full-length compression. In other cases, Class I pantyhose only may be sufficient. These cases include patients with few telangiectasias and no visible inflammatory reaction. However, patients are warned that in cases of excessive skin inflammation, the stockings may need to be replaced with more compressive ones or with compression bandages.

Local and Segmental Compression

When treatment is limited to the lower leg only, below-knee stocking (or bandage) is sufficient. Telangiectasias over a limited area may be treated with local or segmental compression achieved by cotton pads fixed with strips (or full turns) of adhesive bandage, which are kept in place for two to seven days. In selected cases, a compression adhesive, below-knee bandage is applied and kept in place for one or more weeks. An example is the patient with chronic leg edema or dense networks of large telangiectasias on the foot and lower leg. After one or two sessions, the adhesive bandage is replaced by a Class III stocking or removable compression bandage and is worn until the end of treatment.

■ DURATION OF COMPRESSION

Our policy is to maintain daytime compression until all signs of treatment disappear, or for approximately two weeks after the last treatment session. Further compression is advised in cases of hyperpigmentation or telangiectatic matting. Patients treated with a Class III stocking are advised to wear a Class I pantyhose for one or two months after the end of treatment. Patients with widespread or recurrent telangiectasias are advised to use Class I stockings as prophylaxis against further recurrence.

■ FREQUENCY OF SESSIONS

Two to seven days after the first session, the patient is seen to check the response and plan further treatment. It is important not to postpone this examination. Patients who develop an inflammatory reaction with many coagula require prompt evacuation of coagula or modification of the compression regimen to minimize skin pigmentation. If there are many venules to inject, sessions are arranged on a weekly basis, or more often, until all areas have been treated. Many weeks between sessions will not only increase the risk of pigmentation, but may also unnecessarily prolong the treatment. Once a patient's "reaction tendency" is known, most telangiectasias have been damaged, and there are no coagula to evacuate, sessions can be scheduled at two-week intervals or longer.

■ DURATION OF TREATMENT

With the method described in this chapter, a "typical" treatment lasts from one to four months. Such average numbers, however, are a poor guide to predicting the duration of treatment in a single patient. In some cases, sudden destruction of telangiectasias may allow treatment to be completed in one to three sessions, whereas in some cases more than 20 sessions may be needed. Moreover, in some cases, further "touch-up" treatment may be needed 6 to 12 months later. Treatment may be especially prolonged if telangiectatic matting occurs because further injections should not be given until local hyperemia disappears. This can take many months. Unfortunately, all this will be discovered only after treatment has begun and can be an unpleasant surprise for the patient and the doctor.

Long-term results vary. Although some patients may not need further treatment for several years, others need two or more sessions every one or two years to keep their legs in acceptable condition. Occasionally, with congenital widespread telangiectasias (which invariable extend to other parts of the body) or telangiectasias secondary to endocrine, metabolic, or other disease, the patient may be difficult to satisfy. In these cases, realistic treatment goals should be thoroughly discussed prior to treatment. It must be made clear that while it is relatively easy to get rid of many of the worst clusters of telangiectasias, complete clearing of all visible venules may not be achieved. How much one can promise, and achieve, depends not only on the underlying disease, but also on the physician's experience.

◼ REFERENCES

1. Duffy DM: Techniques of small vessel sclerotherapy. In Bergan JJ, Goldman MP, editors: Varicose veins & telangiectasias: diagnosis & treatment. St Louis, 1993, Quality Medical Publishing, Inc.

2. Georgiev M: Post sclerotherapy hyperpigmentations: chromated glycerin as a screen for patients at risk, J Dermatol Surg Oncol 15:204, 1989.

3. Goldman MP, et al.: Sclerosing agents in the treatment of telangiectasias: comparison of clinical and histologic effects of intravascular polidocanol, sodium tetradecyl sulfate, and hypertonic saline in the dorsal rabbit ear vein model, Arch Dermatol 123:1196, 1987.

4. Goldman MP: A comparison of sclerosing agents: clinical and histologic effects of intravenous sodium tetradecyl sulfate and chromated glycerin in the dorsal rabbit ear vein. J Dermatol Surg Oncol 16:18, 1990.

5. Sigg K: Varizen ulcus cruris und thrombose, Berlin, 1976, Springer Verlag.

10

LASER AND NONCOHERENT PULSED LIGHT TREATMENT OF LEG TELANGIECTASIAS AND VENULES

Mitchel P. Goldman

Lasers have been used to treat leg telangiectasia for various reasons. First, lasers have a futuristic appeal. They are perceived as "state of the art" and sought after by the general public because high technology is thought of as safer and better. Lasers have been demonstrated to have theoretical advantages compared with sclerotherapy for treating leg telangiectasia. Sclerotherapy-induced pigmentation is secondary to hemosiderin deposition through extravasated erythrocytes. Laser coagulation of vessels should not have this effect. In the rabbit-ear model, approximately 50% of vessels treated with an effective concentration of sclerosing solution demonstrated extravasated erythrocytes compared with a 30% incidence when treated with the flashlamp pumped pulsed dye laser (FLPDL) (Goldman MP, unpublished observations). Telangiectatic matting (TM) has also not been associated with laser treatment of any vascular condition, but occurs in a significant percentage of sclerotherapy-treated patients. Finally, specific allergenic effects of the sclerosing solution do not occur with laser treatment.

PAST LASER EXPERIENCE

Four types of lasers have been used to treat leg telangiectasias: carbon dioxide, neodymium: yttrium-aluminum-garnet (Nd:YAG), argon, 577-to-585 nm flashlamp pumped pulsed dye (FLPDL), and continuous wave lasers. In addition a novel, noncoherent pulsed light has also been shown to effectively thermocoagulate leg telangiectasia, venules, and reticular veins up to 3 mm in diameter: Photoderm VL light source (Energy Systems Corporation, Newton, MA). Each laser type acts in a different manner to effect vessel destruction. CO_2, Nd:YAG, argon, and continuous wave dye lasers are not entirely specific for vascular tissue due to both wavelength and pulse-durations that are

outside of the thermal relaxation time of the treated vessel. Their energy therefore affects perivascular and cutaneous tissue and causes nonspecific damage. This translates into hypopigmentation and hyperpigmentation and hypertrophic scarring. Thus, although somewhat effective in treating facial vascular abnormalities, these nonspecific lasers are not recommended for treating leg veins.

In addition to ablating the vascular lesion in a specific manner, one must also consider the pathophysiology of the vessels' development. Most abnormal telangiectasias and venules on the leg are derived from venous hypertension. These can arise from arteriovenous malformations or more commonly from larger or more deeply situated veins having valvular incompetence (see Chapter 4). The underlying venous hypertension feeding these vessels must be treated first or the damaged vein will rapidly recanalize.

CURRENT LASERS

Two laser and pulsed-light systems are currently available that specifically affect leg veins without significant adverse sequelae. The FLPDL acts within the thermal relaxation times of blood vessels to produce specific destruction of vessels less than 0.2-mm in diameter. The thermal relaxation time refers to the time it takes for a heated target (in this case the blood vessel wall and endothelium) to dissipate heat. Ideally, one should keep the absorbed thermal energy (heat) within the vessel to prevent unnecessary thermal damage of perivascular structures. The Photoderm VL was developed to treat vessels up to 3 mm in diameter 2 mm beneath the epidermis. However, even with this specificity for treating individual leg veins and telangiectasia, to be successful, high pressure inflow and reflux must first

89

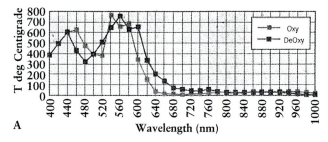

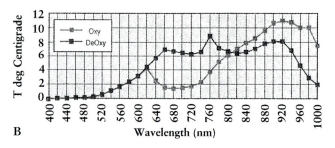

A — Wavelength (nm)

B — Wavelength (nm)

Fig. 10-1. Average temperature increase across a cutaneous vessel as a function of wavelength for two cases: a shallow capillary vessel (similar to those found in a port-wine vascular malformation) and a deeper (2 mm), larger (1 mm) vessel typical of a leg venule. The calculated curves are generated assuming that the main light-absorbing chromophore in the blood is either oxygenated or deoxygenated hemoglobin. The calculation is carried out for a 10J/cm² fluence and does not take into account cooling by heat conductivity. Note the dramatic shift in the optimal wavelength as a function of vessel depth and diameter. Also note the difference between oxygenated and deoxygenated hemoglobin. (Courtesy of Shimon Eckhouse Ph.D., ESC Inc., Newton, MA). (Reproduced with permission from Goldman MP, Fitzpatrick RE: Cutaneous laser surgery. St Louis, 1994, p. 23, Mosby.)

be eliminated. Thus, incompetent perforating veins and junctions (saphenofemoral or saphenopopliteal) or feeding reticular veins must first be treated with sclerotherapy and/or surgery to eliminate venous hypertension into the target vessels.

■ MECHANISM OF ACTION

The main chromophore in the blood vessel is oxyhemoglobin.[1] The oxyhemoglobin absorption spectrum has three major bands calculated for 50 um vessels 0.2 mm deep, the largest at 418 nm and two smaller peaks at 542 and 577 nm. Although there are stronger oxyhemoglobin bands at shorter wavelengths, competing absorption by epidermal melanin overlying the dermal vessels tends to dominate.[2] A restriction of the application of the 577-nm wavelength in treating vascular lesions has been its penetration to only approximately 0.5 mm in depth from the dermal-epidermal junction.[3] However, the depth of vascular damage increases from 0.5 to 1.2 mm by changing the wavelength from 577 to 585 nm while maintaining the same degree of vascular selectivity as for 577-nm irradiation.[4,5] Increasing the wavelength of the FLPDL to 600 nm has also been shown histologically to give deeper thermocoagulation than does a 585 nm FLPDL.[6] Thus, longer wavelengths may be desirable when treating deeper blood vessels (Fig. 10-1).

Besides matching the laser wavelength to the target tissue, it is ideal to limit the laser energy absorption and contain it within the targeted structure. This is accomplished by pulsing the laser. Limiting the duration of laser exposure ensures that highly specific laser energy is delivered in less time than that required for cooling the target vessel, that is, less than the thermal relaxation time.

For superficial cutaneous blood vessels, thermal relaxation times range from 0.1 to 10 ms, depending on the size and type of the vessel,[1,7] and average 1.2 ms.[1] (Table 10-1) In addition to thermal damage produced by the absorption of the 577-nm wavelength, photoacoustic "shock-wave" damage resulting from rapid absorption of energy by the oxyhemoglobin molecules has also been demonstrated.[3,8,9] This shock-wave promotes the undesirable purpuric response commonly seen with the FLPDL, which may take one to three weeks to completely resolve. The advantage of using longer pulse durations that are still within the thermal relaxation times for the targeted blood vessels is that larger diameter blood vessels may be treated. The average diameters of blood vessels in the upper dermis is 40 to 60 um; deeper dermis is 100-400 um, and subcutaneous tissue is 1 to 3 mm. In addition, longer pulses may prevent the shock-wave effect, thus preventing purpura.

Table 10-1 Thermal Relaxation Time of Cutaneous Vessels

Vessel Diameter	Thermal Relaxation Time
20 μm	140 μs
50 μm	1.2 ms
100 μm	3.6 ms
300 μm	5–10 ms

■ LASER TESTING AND RESULTS

We systematically examined the clinical effects of various powers of the FLPDL in specific leg telangiectasias. We chose type 1 red telangiectasias less than 0.2 mm in diameter and vessels arising as a function of telangiectatic matting for examination because these vessels are the most difficult to treat with standard sclerotherapy techniques.[9,10] The FLPDL produces vascular injury in a histologic pattern that is different than that produced by sclerotherapy: less extravasation of red blood cells, decreased perivascular inflammation, and the production of intravascular fibrin strands. This may translate into a decreased incidence or extent of postsclerosis pigmentation and a decreased incidence or extent of telangiectatic matting.

Patients with red-leg telangiectasias less than 0.2 mm in diameter were treated with a Candela FLPDL tuned to 585 nm with a pulse duration of 450 μs at energies ranging from 6.0 to 8.5 J/cm^2 delivered through a 5-mm spot size to the entire length of the telangiectasia. The most significant outcome of FLPDL treatment of leg telangiectasias was the relative lack of adverse sequelae and complications. With FLPDL treatment alone, there were no episodes of telangiectatic matting in the 101 treated sites. (As of this writing we have treated more than 1,000 sites of leg telangiectasia with still no evidence of telangiectatic matting or complications other than described below.) All patients with hyperpigmentation induced by FLPDL experienced complete resolution within four months (Fig. 10-2). There were no episodes of cutaneous ulceration, thrombophlebitis, or other complications.

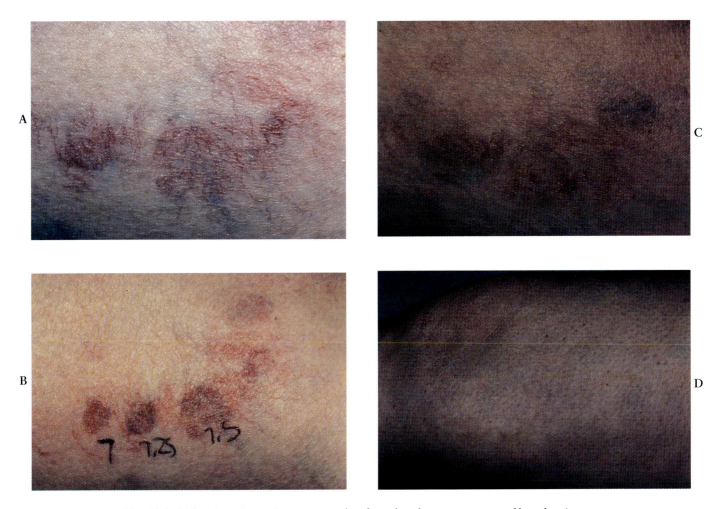

Fig. 10-2. Telangiectatic matting nine months after sclerotherapy treatment of leg telangiectasia on the medial thigh. **A,** Immediately before treatment. **B,** Immediately after laser impacts were performed at the indicated energies in J/cm^2, nine 5-mm impacts were given at each test dose. **C,** Two months after tests, some hyperpigmentation is noted. **D,** One year after treatment of the entire area at 7.25 J/cm^2, there is completely resolution. (Reproduced with permission from Goldman MP: Sclerotherapy treatment of varicose and telangiectatic leg veins, ed 2. St Louis, 1995, Mosby.)

The most effective laser energy is between 7.0 and 8.0 J/cm². At these laser parameters, 48% to 67% of telangiectatic patches totally fade within four months. The percentage of telangiectasias that totally fade increases when only vessels without reticular feeding veins are considered. There appears to be no difference in the response to PDL in telangiectatic matting vessels.

■ PHOTODERM VL LIGHT SOURCE

An ideal laser or pulsed light source to treat leg veins should have a wavelength that can penetrate to the full depth of the target blood vessel and deliver sufficient energy to the target vessel to thermocoagulate the entire vessel wall without damaging perivascular tissues or overlying skin. In addition, the energy should be delivered without causing a shock-wave to prevent posttreatment purpura. To maximize efficacy in treating leg veins a novel pulsed light source has been developed. This new technology is more appropriate for leg telangiectasias and venules because these vessels are substantially larger, are more deeply situated in the skin, and have thicker walls.

To treat larger vessels, energy must be delivered in the range of approximately 3 to 30 ms pulses so absorbed heat from erythrocytes has time to diffuse throughout the vessel circumference. This can require double or triple simultaneous pulses to maximize absorption of light fluence to the vessel while allowing thermal cooling of epidermal and perivascular tissues (Fig. 10-3). To treat deep vascular structures the wave-

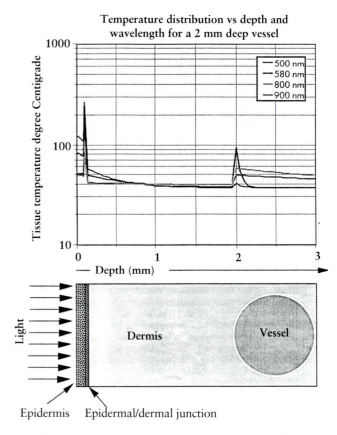

Fig. 10-4. Temperature distribution across skin and blood vessel. A 2 mm deep, 1 mm diameter vessel is assumed. A 10 J/cm² fluence is assumed at four different wavelengths. The calculation takes into account scattering effects in the epidermis and dermis and fluence enhancement caused by scattering. Note the very high temperature on the skin surface and at the epidermal and dermal junction and shallow penetration for the shorter wavelengths. (Courtesy of Shimon Eckhouse, Ph.D., ESC Inc., Newton, MA) (Reproduced with permission from Goldman MP, Fitzpatrick RE: Cutaneous laser surgery. St Louis, 1994, p. 29, Mosby.)

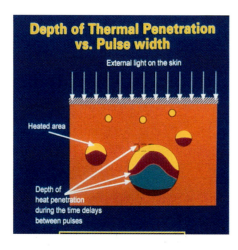

Fig. 10-3. Schematic diagram of the effect of repetitive pulses of the Photoderm light source on a 2 mm vessel 1 mm below the epidermis. (Courtesy of Shimon Eckouse, Ph.D., Energy Systems Corporation, Newton, MA). (Reproduced with permission from Goldman MP: Sclerotherapy treatment of varicose and telangiectatic leg veins, ed 2, St Louis, 1995, Mosby.)

length must be long enough to reach not only the top of the vessel beneath the skin, but also the entire diameter of the vessel (Fig. 10-4). A longer wavelength will also minimize coupling to the epidermis with resulting heat absorption. Finally, because leg telangiectasias and venules have thicker walls than the ectatic vessels of port-wine vascular malformations, higher energy fluences must be given.

Fortunately, calculated energy absorption for oxygenated and deoxygenated hemoglobin is very different for vessels 1 mm in diameter and 2 mm beneath the dermal-epidermal junction (see Fig. 10-1). In these deeper and larger vessels, oxygenated hemoglobin peaks at 920 nm and deoxygenated hemoglobin has a fairly plateau peak between 660 and 920nm. Thus,

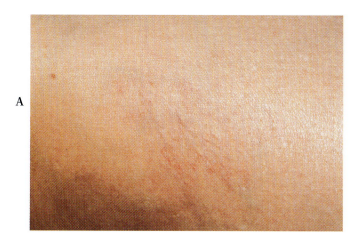
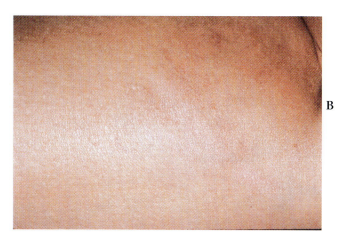

Fig. 10-5. Clinical appearance of telangiectasia on the thigh of a 32-year-old woman. A, Before treatment. B, Clinical appearance 10 weeks after treatment. (Reproduced with permission from Goldman MP: Sclerotherapy treatment of varicose and telangiectatic leg veins, ed 2, St Louis, 1995, Mosby.)

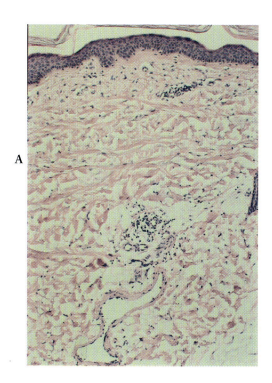
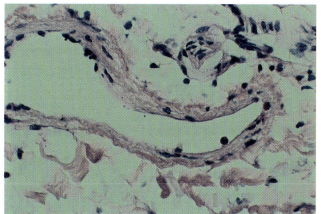
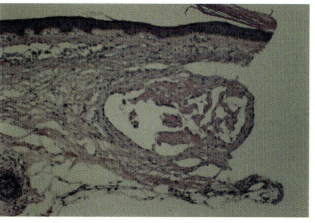

Fig. 10-6. Appearance of venule 1 mm in diameter stained with hematoxylin-eosin 48 hours after treatment with the Photoderm VL at 26 J/cm² delivered in a double pulse 6 ms and 15 ms long separated by 50 ms. **A,** Note size and depth of vessel that appears collapsed from biopsy and processing artifact, but devoid of blood, original magnification ×50. **B,** same vessel as in A. Note intravascular margination of mast cell and lymphocytes with partial destruction of endothelium and vessel wall, original magnification ×200. **C,** 2-mm diameter vessel, 3 weeks after treatment with Photoderm VL. Note reorganizing thrombosis. H & E × 50. (A and B reproduced with permission from Goldman MP: Sclerotherapy treatment of varicose and telangiectatic leg veins, ed 2, St Louis, 1995, Mosby.)

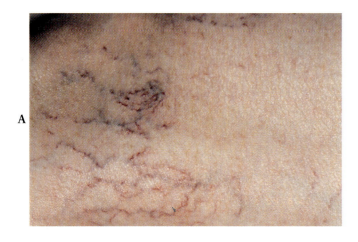

A

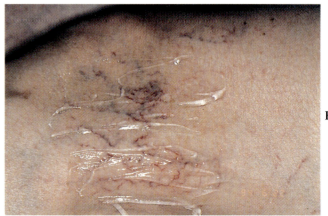

B

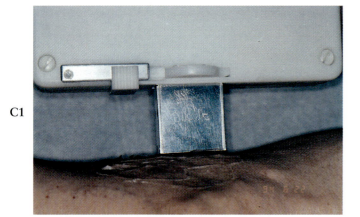

C1

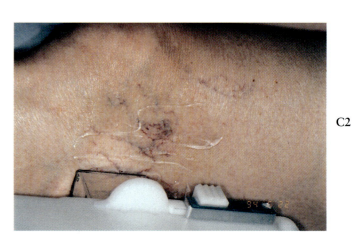

C2

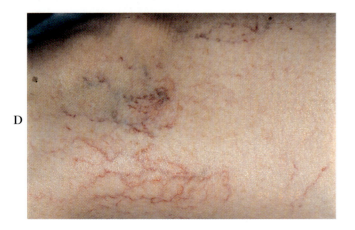

D

Fig. 10-7. Photoderm VL treatment. **A,** Appearance of telangiectasia 0.4–0.6 mm diameter on the inner thigh before treatment. **B,** Application of clear coupling gel. **C1** and **C2,** Position of photoderm light-guide on telangiectasia. **D,** Appearance immediately after treatment. Note mild urtication and erythemia without purpura of treated area.

using a light source between 600 and 900 mm has the advantage of both penetrating to the proper depth of leg telangiectasias and venules and being selectively absorbed by oxygenated-deoxygenated hemoglobin.

The Photoderm VL can deliver energy fluences of 20 to 80 J/cm^2 over 2 to 20 ms and can be repetitively pulsed with delays between pulses of 50 to 1,000 ms. This has been demonstrated to effectively thermocoagulate vessels up to 3 mm in diameter 2 mm below the dermal-epidermal junction as well as telangiectasia 0.2 to 0.6 mm in diameter (Fig. 10-5).

Histologic evaluation demonstrates that the Photoderm VL does not cause vessel rupture as is also evident by the lack of clinical purpura. Instead, the vessel wall is more slowly heated, producing destruction (Fig. 10-6).

The Photoderm VL delivers its energy through a "footprint" whose size and dimensions can vary based on the requirements of the target vessel. The present machine has a standard footprint or spot size of 8 mm × 35 mm. This permits efficient treatment of large sections of vessels.

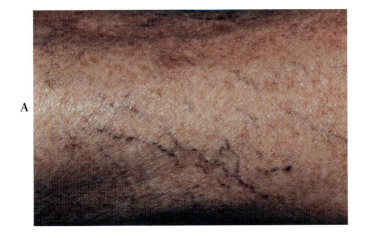

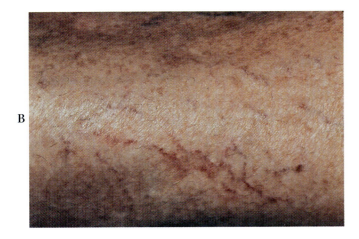

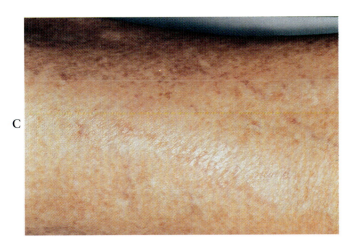

Fig. 10-8. A, Clinical appearance of 0.6mm diameter vessels before treatment. **B,** Immediately after treatment. **C,** Ten weeks after treatment, complete resolution has occurred without adverse sequellae.

PREVENTING THERMAL INJURY

To prevent nonspecific damage to overlying skin, clear thermal coupling gel is placed on the skin as a layer between the flashlamp window and epidermis. The gel acts as a heat sink, absorbing reflected photons from the epidermis to prevent epidermal heating. We have found that the gel needs to be changed every 5 to 10 pulses depending on the delivered energy fluence. When a thin layer of gel is spread over the entire treatment area, the gel usually needs to be changed once or twice during a treatment session (Figs. 10-7 and 10-8).

At this writing, the Photoderm VL is in its final stages of development. Vessels up to 3 mm in diameter have been successfully obliterated without significant adverse sequelae. Patients report less pain compared with the FLPDL, and treatment sessions are well tolerated. The only adverse effects noted are slight epidermal burning without resulting scarring in patients with pigmented skin Fitzpatrick type 3 or greater. In addition, intradermal nevi, lentigines, and other pigmented lesions within the treated area disappear after treatment.

CONCLUSIONS

Laser or pulsed-light treatment of leg veins has the advantage of being relatively noninvasive (no needles) and nontoxic (no injection of sclerosing solution). Decreased inflammation also prevents the development of telangiectatic matting. Complete thermocoagulation prevents extravasation of red-blood cells that limits posttreatment hyperpigmentation. However, high pressure reflux from incompetent perforator, reticular, or varicose veins must first be treated either surgically or with sclerotherapy before laser or photothermocoagulation can be expected to be effective.

■ REFERENCES

1. Anderson RR, Parrish JA: Microvasculature can be selectively damaged using dye lasers: a basic theory and experimental evidence in human skin, Lasers Surg Med 1:263, 1981.

2. van Gemert MJC, Welch AJ, Amin AP: Is there an optimal laser treatment for port-wine stains? Lasers Surg Med 6:76, 1986.

3. Nakagawa H, Tan OT, Parrish JA: Ultrastructural changes in human skin after exposure to a pulsed laser, J Invest Dermatol 84:396, 1985.

4. Tan OT, Murray S, Kurban AK: Action spectrum of vascular specific injury using pulsed irradiation, J Invest Dermatol 92:868, 1989.

5. Anderson R, Parrish JA: The optics of human skin, J Invest Dermatol 77:13, 1981.

6. Goldman L, Kerr JH, Larkin M, et al.: 600 nm flash pumped dye laser for fragile telangiectasia of the elderly, Las Surg Med 13:227-233, 1993.

7. Anderson RR, Parrish JA: Selective photothermolysis: precise microsurgery by selective absorption of pulsed radiation, Science 220:524, 1983.

8. Gange RW et al.: Effect of preirradiation tissue target temperature upon selective vascular damage induced by 577-nm tunable dye laser pulses, Microvasc Res 28:125, 1980.

9. Goldman MP et al.: Pulsed-dye laser treatment of telangiectases with and without sub-therapeutic sclerotherapy: clinical and histologic examination of the rabbit ear vein model, J Am Acad Dermatol 23:23, 1990.

10. Goldman MP, Fitzpatrick RE: Pulsed-dye laser treatment of leg telangiectasia: with and without simultaneous sclerotherapy, J Dermatol Surg Oncol 16:338, 1990.

Part III

Macrosclerotherapy

11

INJECTION SCLEROTHERAPY FOR VARICOSE VEINS—A VIEW FROM IRELAND

Mary Henry

Some 35 years ago the injection treatment of varicose veins known as compression sclerotherapy (CS) was developed in Dublin by Professor W.G. Fegan.[1] The treatment involves the diagnosis and then injection of specific sites in the superficial venous complex. These sites control filling of the superficial venous system when the patient moves from lying to standing upright.

The "empty vein" technique is used when the injections are given. The whole leg is bandaged with compression bandages, and extra compression is applied to the injection sites. After treatment, immediately walking is required to prevent the development of superficial phlebitis and should be continued on a daily basis throughout the course of CS.

Essentially the treatment aims at restoring the pumping capacity of the muscle pumps in the foot, calf, and thigh, rather than the eradication of all superficial varices. An improvement in the proximal veins can be seen when the distal veins are treated,[2] therefore the most distal "leaks" from the deep to the superficial system are treated first.

Patients who are referred to a varicose-vein clinic with varicose veins often have signs and symptoms indicating that their problems are caused by other medical conditions. Diagnosis and treatment of the coexisting condition is essential and often preferable before treatment of the venous condition commences.

The most common coexisting medical conditions are orthopadic and arterial, therefore the patient's symptoms can be exacerbated by treating their venous condition first. Extra walking can cause increased pain in patients with orthopadic problems, and tight bandaging may be strongly contraindicated in arterial disease. Edema may be symptomatic of systemic disease and not of venous insufficiency, and care must be taken to diagnose the cause of ulcers that are nonvaricose.

Most patients can be treated once a diagnosis of venous insufficiency as a cause of the patient's signs and symptoms has been made. Some practitioners reserve CS as a finale to operative treatment,[3] however, this ensures that the patient has endured the worst aspects of both forms of treatment.

An anesthetic with a hospital stay and an operation that can result in the patient having scars, followed by a length of time in bandages, is the major disadvantage for the patient being treated by CS.

Although the risk of recurrence may be higher following CS, it is important to remember that those patients who opt for CS would prefer the risk of recurrence rather than undergo operative treatment. When the saphenofemoral junction is incompetent, results are least satisfactory.[4] Doppler examination will confirm whether the valve is competent or not. A flush-tie ligation before treatment can be performed, but it should be explained to the patient that this procedure is not a "cure all." In many patients when the saphenofemoral junction has been tied, varicose veins recur.[5]

An absolute contraindication to injection treatment is the inability to walk. The presence of ulcers or eczema is not a contraindication; neither is a history of a deep-vein thrombosis or superficial phlebitis, but this should be carefully noted in the medical history. If the patient is allergic to one sclerosant, then another should be used. Compression is more difficult to obtain in patients who have obese legs, and treatment should not be attempted above the midthigh.

Pregnant patients can be treated,[6] but this is recommended early in the pregnancy because in later months walking may be too tiring. Patients who require treatment of superficial veins for cosmetic reasons only should be informed, before commencing treatment, that occasionally some staining can occur at the injection sites. If treatment is to be carried out in a country with a hot climate, it is better to wait until the coolest time of the year because the bandages and elastic stockings could be very uncomfortable in hot weather. There is a slightly increased risk of thrombophlebitis in patients taking oral contraceptive pills, and therefore they should be advised to stop taking the pills for a few weeks before treatment and not to recommence until treatment has been completed. There do not appear to be any problems in patients who are taking hormone-replacement therapy.

MATERIALS AND METHODS

It is essential that special clinics be set up specifically for injection compression sclerotherapy treatment and that this treatment be carried out by a trained practitioner. Patients' charts should have extensive personal details. Age, parity, job description, and a family history of varicose veins can be important when the physician is deciding and advising on treatment. Some older patients, who have not been very active, should be advised to practice the required amount of walking before treatment commences. Women who have not completed their families should be advised regarding the possibility of recurrence with further pregnancies. Patients with standing jobs should be informed that their occupations are important factors in developing venous disease.[7]

Coexisting medical conditions and current medication must be noted, and details of blood pressure, urinalysis, and blood counts should be taken. Any past history of allergies should be recorded, as should previous illnesses and any past operations. A past history of a deep-vein thrombosis or pulmonary embolism and any previous treatment for varicose veins either by CS or operation is most important and should be carefully documented.

A sketch of both legs should be made on the chart, from both an anterior and a posterior aspect. All obvious venous complexes should be filled in, ulcers noted, and any scars from previous operations noted. The sites of any injection given should be recorded on this sketch at each visit. If easily available, photographs of the patient's legs, taken at the first visit may be useful. The chart must have space for notes to be made of the number of injections given, the progress of treatment as assessed by the doctor, and comments made by the patient.

Two milliliter disposable syringes and 25-gauge disposable needles with a clear shank are used. The clear shank allows the doctor to know immediately when the vein has been entered. The sclerosant used is % sodium tetradecyl sulphate (STS). Other sclerosants should be used if the patient has had a previous allergic reaction. Four-inch cotton-crepe bandages are used to

apply compression to the whole leg. Shaped sorbo rubber pads are used to produce extra compression over the injection site. Adhesive bandages, nonallergic if possible, are used to keep the cotton-crepe bandages in place. Elastic stockings may be worn over the bandages to give further compression, and dressings for eczema or ulcers will be needed.

TECHNIQUE OF COMPRESSION SCLEROTHERAPY

After standing on a low stool for a couple of minutes to allow the venous complexes to fill, the patient is examined. All visible veins are marked using a skin pencil (Fig. 11-1). The leg is palpated, and any further veins that can be felt are also marked. Percussion of a large vein will often reveal further veins that were not visible. The extent of the varicose complexes should then be obvious.

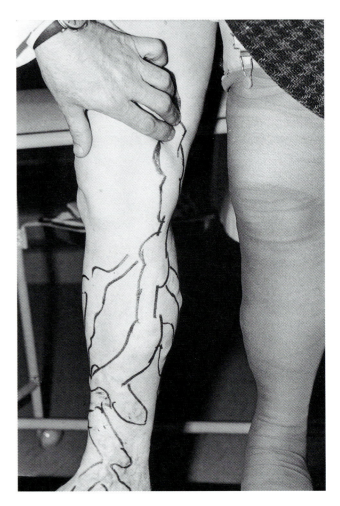

Fig. 11-1. A skin pencil is used to mark all those visible venous complexes.

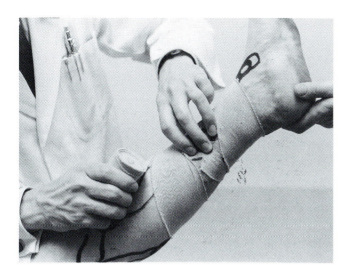

Fig. 11-2. With the leg raised, orifices in the deep fascia can be felt.

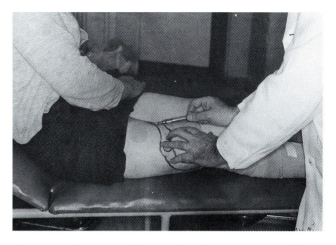

Fig. 11-3. Starting at the most distal site 0.5 to 1 cc of sclerosant is injected.

The patient sits on the couch and lies back with the legs hanging over the end of the couch. The limb under examination is raised, and, with the muscles relaxed, the leg is palpated. With the leg in this position, orifices in the deep fascia can be felt (Fig. 11-2). These orifices should be marked; they are often the sites that control filling of the superficial venous complexes.

A further test is carried out to see if these are the points from which filling of the superficial venous complexes takes place. As many of these sites as possible are compressed by the doctor's fingers. The patient is then asked to stand and with the compression maintained, the doctor watches for filling of the superficial complexes. The test is repeated until the sites that prevent filling are discovered.

Following selection of the sites to be injected the patient sits on a couch with legs extended. Starting at the most distal site, an injection of 0.5 to 1 cc of sclerosant is made (Fig. 11-3) after raising the patient's leg to chest height, to empty the vein, and with a finger above and below the injection site to isolate the segment. It is only necessary to inject the sites where digital pressure has controlled filling of the superficial complexes. It is not necessary to give multiple injections along the vein.

A bandage is applied on either side of the injected area and then over it, and a compression pad is bandaged into place over the injection site (Fig. 11-4.) The technique of bandaging should be learned by all clinicians because it plays such an important role in the injection treatment.[8] Further injections are given, with the physician working proximally. The whole limb should be bandaged from the root of the toes to a few inches above the highest injection site.

An adhesive bandage is applied to the skin at the top of the bandages to hold them in place and can be applied down the leg for added security (Fig. 11-5). Following treatment the patient must walk immediately for one hour. If travel for a long distance after treatment is necessary, the patient should be advised to stop about every hour and walk for five minutes.

On the days following treatment the patient should walk for an hour every day and should avoid standing. This prevents superficial phlebitis, encourages the development of the muscle pumps and prevents the formation of edema.

About two weeks after treatment the patient returns to the clinic, the bandages are cut off, and the leg is reexamined with the patient in the standing position. Edema, which may have been present at the first visit examination, is usually much improved after bandaging and walking.

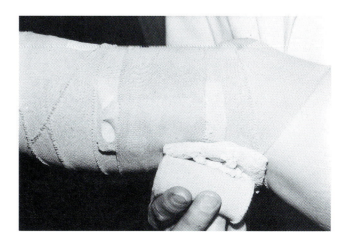

Fig. 11-4. After one turn of bandage a compression pad is bandaged into place.

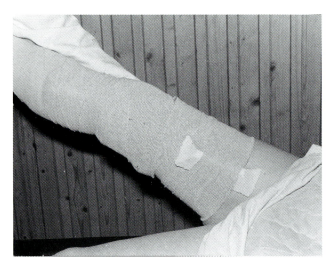

Fig. 11-5. An adhesive bandage is applied to the skin at the top of the bandages and down the leg for added security.

The injection sites are examined. A short cordlike segment of vein is the ideal result. At this stage the area may still feel tender. Filling some of the superficial complexes of varicose veins can still take place if all the sites that require injection have not been treated. These sites should now be injected, the leg rebandaged as before, and the patient advised to continued walking.

The patient's leg should remain bandaged until the injection sites are painless. This usually takes three to four weeks, but longer may be necessary in patients who had very extensive varices. Reddy and associates[9] found no significant difference in the results of treatment following bandaging for more than three weeks.

Patients are advised to wear elastic stockings for four to six weeks after the bandages are removed. For patients who work in standing occupations, wearing an elastic stocking is often advisable to prevent the development of further varicose veins.

If any further varicose veins develop or recur, further courses of treatment are quite possible some years later. This is most likely in patients who have standing occupations, further pregnancies, or a strong family history of varicose veins.[10]

■ SIMULTANEOUS TREATMENT OF ULCERS

The presence of a varicose ulcer does not prevent treating the patient's varicose veins. On the contrary, treating the veins usually leads to more rapid healing of the ulcer.[11] Care should be taken, however, not to inject areas of cellulitis. If cellulitis is present, systemic antibiotics are required.

Local treatment of ulcers with antibiotic creams or powders is not advisable as this can led to the development of allergies to the antibiotic. A growth of mixed organisms is present on most ulcers and a month's treatment with the appropriate antibiotics can increase the rate of healing.[12] Numerous local treatments can be used, but the treatment of the patient's underlying venous problem is much more important. Often veins very close to the ulcer site must be injected to heal the ulcer. Excessive cleaning of ulcers can destroy new epithelial tissue, as can too-frequent dressing. Although the patient's comfort is of primary importance, it must be stressed that frequent dressing may be more harmful than helpful.

Varicose eczema should be treated by applying creams containing low-dose corticosteroids and usually improves within a few days when treatment of the veins is started. Antihistamines may be required by some patients who have severe itching. Many patients have very dry skin, and they should be encouraged to apply emollient cream to the skin after treatment. Creams containing corticosteroids should not be applied around the ulcers because healing will be delayed. Using disinfectant in the bath is discouraged because it is counterproductive.

■ COMPLICATIONS

Anaphylactic reaction to the sclerosant used can occur, and the doctor should have the facilities available to treat this complication. The immediate administration of intravenous hydrocortisone is adequate in most cases, but adrenaline and oxygen should be available.

Fortunately it occurs rarely with STS, but if a reaction does occur, an alternative sclerosant must be used to treat such patients subsequently.

Occasionally a general allergic rash occurs about one hour after treatment. This responds readily to antihistamines, and a different sclerosant should be used for further injections.

Extra vascular injection of a sclerosant, particularly if it is close to the skin, can cause tissue necrosis. The resultant ulcers can be very slow to heal and can leave a scar. There appears to be little difference in the healing rate of whichever local application is used.

Inadvertent arterial injection is a serious complication. The most vulnerable artery is the posterior tibial artery behind the medial malleolus. Immediate action should be taken to reduce the amount of tissue damage. The foot should be cooled with ice, localized intraarterial heparin administered, and intravenous heparinization commenced. The patient should be admitted to hospital where the intervention of a vascular surgeon may be necessary.

Inadequate compression at injection sites allows superficial phlebitis to develop. This can also develop in the long saphenous vein if the sharp edge of bandage cuts into the vein. A pad bandaged into place over the long saphenous vein will prevent this complication. It is most important that the patient walks immediately after treatment to prevent the development of superficial phlebitis.

Pain or numbness in the area of distribution of a superficial nerve can occur if, inadvertently, an injection damages a nerve. Pressure from the bandage around the head of the fibule on the peroneal nerve can do the same. The damage is usually transitory, and the patient can be reassured that full recovery of sensation will take place.

Brown pigmentation at injection sites can take place, and the patient should be warned about this, particularly if treatment is being sought for cosmetic reasons only.

Occasionally a painful intravenous hematoma can occur at an injection site. Usually this occurs where the injected vein is large, and compression has been inadequate. The hematoma will resolve spontaneously, but it can be aspirated using a wide-bore needle; a incision is unnecessary. Firm compression should be reapplied until the area is no longer tender. Brown pigmentation can occur at the site.

Occasionally an allergy to the crepe bandage can occur, which will be diagnosed by the classic extension of eczema in the area covered by the bandage. This can be counteracted by putting Redigauze under the bandage.

RESULTS

Any patient with a family history of varicose veins is particularly liable to recurrence or to new varices, as are those in standing occupations.[7] Therefore it is important that elastic stockings or elastic tights are prescribed on a long-term basis.[13]

Simultaneous injection treatment in patients with varicose ulcers has a cure rate of almost 80%.[11] This compares favorably with other forms of treatment.[14]

Controversy has continued as to whether injection treatment or surgery is the better form of treatment for varicose veins. Hoerdegan and Sigg[15] concluded that both treatments gave similarly good results and advocated that an alternative to operative treatment involving a simple painless procedure should be offered to the patient enabling no loss of working hours. This alternative treatment has been shown to be more economical.[16]

It is difficult to know whether new veins develop or old ones recur, however, the importance of follow-up cannot be over emphasized,[17] and therefore patients should be reviewed at three months, six months, and one year depending on the extent of treatment and thereafter at yearly intervals.

REFERENCES

1. Fegan WG: Continuous compression technique of injecting varicose veins, Lancet 2:109, 1963.
2. Quill RD, Fegan WG: Reversibility of femorosaphenous reflux, Br J Surg 58:5, 197?.
3. Hobbs JT: Surgery and sclerotherapy in the treatment of varicose veins, Arch Surg 90:793-796, 1974.
4. Hobbs JT: The treatment of varicose veins, Br J Surg 55:777, 1968.
5. Sheppard M: A procedure for the prevention of recurrent saphenofemoral incompetence, Aust NZ J Surg 48:322-326, 1978.
6. Fegan WG, Pegum JM: The treatment of varicose veins in pregnancy, Ob/Gyn Digest 8:59, 1966.
7. Askar O, Emera A: Varicose veins and occupation. J Egypt Med Assoc 53:34-349, 1970.
8. Gundersen J: Bandaging of the lower leg, Phlebology 7:50-53, 1992.
9. Reddy P, Wickers J, Terry T, Lamont P, Moller J, Dormandy JA: What is the correct period of bandaging following sclerotherapy? Phlebology :27, 1986.
10. Henry M, Corless C: The incidence of varicose veins in Ireland, Phlebology 4:33, 1989.
11. Dinn E, Henry M: Treatment of venous ulceration by injection sclerotherapy and compression hosiery: a 5-year study, Phlebology 7:23-26, 1992.
12. Schraibman I: The bacteriology of leg ulcers, Phlebology 2:265, 1987.
13. Dinn E, Henry M: Value of light weight elastic tights in standing occupations, Phlebology 4:45-49, 1989.
14. Akasson H: Long term clinical results following correction of incompetent superficial and perforating veins in patients with deep venous incompetence and ulcers, Phlebology 8:28-3, 1993.
15. Hoerdegen K, Sigg K: Injection-compression sclerotherapy of the greater saphenous vein with proximal incompetence (crosse insufficiency) as an alternative to surgery, Phlebology 3:4-48, 1988.
16. Piachaud D, Weddell JM: The cost of treating varicose veins, Lancet 2:9-92, 1972.
17. Juhan C, Haupert S, Miltgen G, Barthelemy P, and Eklof B: Recurrent varicose veins, Phlebology 5:20-2, 1990.

12

MACROSCLEROTHERAPY AND COMPRESSION

Richard J. Tazelaar and H.A. Martino Neumann

Compression therapy is one of the most important therapy modalities available for the phlebologist. It can be used either alone or as part of sclerotherapy, surgery, or any other treatment for venous diseases. Several complications from other therapies as well as from the underlying disease, such as phlebitis, allergic contact dermatitis, hospitalization, and incapacity for work can be avoided by using compression therapy. Compression therapy is only of great value when combined with the function of the muscle pumps of which the calf-muscle pump is the most important.

The term "ambulant compression" is used to emphasize the close relationship between bandage and muscle-pump activity. The active-muscle pump combined with the pressure of the bandage or stocking on vessels and subcutaneous tissue is responsible for the effect of compression therapy. Recently, compression therapy was reviewed by the authors.[1]

■ AIM AND MECHANISM OF COMPRESSION THERAPY

The venous system is, more than any other "vessel system," affected by compression therapy. Epifascial and subfascial veins are compressed as documented by Doppler, duplex, and phlebography. Thrombi, if present, are fixed against the vessel wall. Even incompetent perforator veins can be compressed by using special pelottes. This results in at least a partial correction of the reflux and diminishing of the venous volume. When the venous volume is decreased with compression, the muscle pump becomes more effective. Venous flow velocity increases, which prevents thrombophlebitis and deep-vein thrombosis.[2] In a well-performed, five-year follow-up study, adequate com-

pression therapy was proved to prevent 50% of the postthrombotic syndrome.[3]

Compression therapy also influences microcirculation. This is of special interest because the microcirculatory alterations induced by venous insufficiency are responsible for the skin changes that occur in venous insufficiency syndrome, including the venous leg ulcer. Compression therapy increases tissue pressure, but deceases postcapillary pressure and filtration. Absorption increases in addition to lymph drainage. Edema, synthesis of collagen I and III, which results in dermatoliposclerosis and formation of collagen IV in the capillaries, decreases. Velocity in the capillaries increases, which prevents microthrombosis and white-cell trapping.[8]

Well-performed compression therapy will not significantly influence arterial inflow. Skin circulation will be reduced, especially by the resting pressure of the bandage. This resting pressure is high compared to nonelastic bandages. As a consequence of the elasticity, the risk for ischemia and necrosis is much higher when using elastic bandages rather than nonelastic bandages. However, in experienced hands, compression therapy can be used with great success.[2]

■ AIM AND MECHANISM OF SCLEROTHERAPY

The medical aim in treating varicose veins is to eliminate reflux in the venous system to reestablish a normal microcirculatory pressure profile. Sclerotherapy is widely used with or without selective surgery for treating varicose veins. With sclerotherapy, endofibrosis obliterates perforating veins and transforms varicose veins into a fibrotic cord.[5,6] Large thrombi have to be avoided to minimize periphlebitis, recanalization, and pigmentation. Although these thrombi can easily be removed by small incisions and manual compression, better results are obtained if this is step is not necessary.

Combination of Compression and Sclerotherapy

Although in the classical French School of Tournay no compression was used at all, not even for sclerosing the saphenous vein,[6] today most physicians use the combination of injection/sclerotherapy and compression. For this reason it is better to talk about "sclerocompression therapy." In our opinion it is essential to combine sclerotherapy with compression therapy.

By compressing the insufficient perforator and increasing venous flow, leakage of the sclerosing agent into the deep system will be minimized. This explains the rarity of deep-venous thrombosis after sclerocompression therapy compared with sclerotherapy alone. With uncomplicated varicose veins the influence of compression therapy on the calf-muscle pump is minimal.[7] This effect increases when venous insufficiency is more severe. The most important mechanism of compression therapy in sclerocompression therapy, however, is to bring the venous walls close together, minimizing thrombus formation.

Amount of Pressure

The amount of pressure depends on the intravascular pressure of the treated vein and the pressure of the surrounding tissue. With the patient in the supine position, a pressure of approximately 30 mmHg is sufficient to collapse all superficial veins.[2] Van Cleef demonstrated by angiography narrowing of the longitudinal veins in the supine position with pressures below 20 mmHg.[8] However, reflux still exists when an intercorneal space at valve commissures is involved. In a special vein model, a volume reduction of 94% can be demonstrated with a pressure of 54 mmHg. Depending on the size and shape of a pelotte, according to Laplace law, less bandage pressure is required to obtain the same result.[8,9] As shown by duplex scanning, a medium pressure of 89 mmHg is necessary to occlude the greater saphenous vein when the patient is standing. Reflux is abolished in 8 of 19 patients at a medium pressure of 31 mmHg.[11] We have to keep in mind that all these studies are static and that the pressure in the venous system is affected by the characteristics of the type of compression bandage and the intravenous pressure profile.

Duration of Compression

How long should compression continue to give optimal results? From a histological study, Fegan indicates that at least six weeks are required for endofibrosis to occur.[5] Since elastic bandages lose their effective pressures after six to eight hours,[12] several types of elastic bandages and various durations of compression have been developed. Similar results have been noticed after compression for three days, one week, three weeks, and six weeks.[13-15] However, the follow-up in these studies is restricted to three months[14] with a maximum of two years.[13] Special attention was paid to subjective symptoms, the extent of remaining varicose veins, and phlebitis. It is remarkable that a quarter of the patients from the group with three weeks of compression, as well as the group with six weeks of compression, have phlebitis after three months. This seems unacceptably high.

Our Own Approach to Sclerocompression Therapy

We prefer to eliminate the major sources of reflux by selective surgery. Pretreatment investigations include clinical history, physical examination, and noninvasive examination. In most cases, photoplethysmography in combination with Doppler ultrasound is sufficient to develop an individual therapeutical strategy.[16] Ligation of an incompetent perforator vein or ligation of the saphenofemoral and/or saphenopopliteal junction (so-called crosse-ectomy), whether or not in combination with short stripping of the greater saphenous vein, is our preferred method of selective surgery. All other varicose veins are treated with sclerocompression therapy or phlebectomy according to Muller. In a practice of more than ten years, we have studied several types of bandages and duration of compression and have developed a method that appears to be satisfactory.

Only a small amount of blood is left in the varicose vein ("empty vein technique"). This can be achieved by injecting the leg when the patient is in the horizontal or even the Trendelenburg position. If necessary, the varicose vein can be stroked empty. The distance between injections is short (3 to 5 cm), and the volume of the sclerosing agent restricted to 0.2 to 0.3 cc. A larger dose may be required (0.5 cc) for an insufficient perforating vein. The sclerosant concentration has to be correct, depending on the amount of reflux and the tortuosity of the varicose vein. A concentration that is too weak results in insufficient endofibrosis, and a concentration too strong leads to an excessive inflammatory reaction.[15] Accurate compression over the entire length of the varicose vein is desired to keep the thrombus small and to secure it to the vessel wall. If one of these conditions has not been fulfilled, a larger thrombus may arise or a part of the varicose veins may not fibrose.

Compression therapy, as we use it, has two components. The first is continuous compression, day and night. This is placed over the varicose veins by using special pelottes. These consist of very tightly twisted and firmly compressible rolls of cotton wool with a diameter of ± 2 cm. Contrary to the often used pelottes exclusively placed upon the points of injection, we fix the rolls of cotton wool over the entire course of the varicose veins, following the curves accurately. Intravasal accumulations of blood are prevented, provided that the injections are given with sufficient distance in between. The pelottes are secured with nonelastic plaster material (FixomullR). When the direct surroundings mainly consist of subcutaneous fat, as is the case on the upper leg, the cotton wool submerges almost completely. According to Laplace law, a high compression (> 70 mmHg) occurs just beneath the pelotte. (Recent observations were obtained with the Oxford Pressure Measurement Instrument, to be published soon).

The pelottes stay in place for several days to two weeks. On bony parts, we use less tightly twisted rolls. On top of the secured, cotton-wool rolls, two elastic stockings are worn: a Class I stocking day and night, and on top of that a Class II stocking worn during the daytime. The pressure of two stockings worn on top of one another is complementary. A Class I stocking with a pressure of 12 to 18 mmHg around the ankle (also in horizontal position) does not disturb the arterial circulation. A Class II stocking worn on top of that during the daytime gives an extra pressure of ± 30 mmHg so an ankle pressure of ± 40 to 45 mmHg is reached. This pressure combined with the pelotte is sufficient.

We use elastic stockings instead of elastic bandages because they are easy to handle and do not have to be renewed during the different sclerocompression treatment sessions, which saves money. Moreover, elastic stockings prevent slipping even on very fat thighs, so the pressure decline is much smaller. The stockings also fix the pelottes and put extra pressure on the skin under the pelotte. The more serious the venous insufficiency, the more important the effects on the muscle pump.[7]

When the pelottes are removed, the Class I stocking will not be worn anymore. Depending on the amount of reflux before treatment and the size of the varicose veins, the Class II stockings will be worn for one to four weeks during the daytime. For example, on reticular varicose veins, the pelottes are removed after five to seven days, and for one more week a complementary Class II stocking is worn. On an insufficient

perforating vein with much more reflux after treatment, the pelottes are not removed until after two to three weeks, and the Class II stocking is worn for three to four more weeks. The practical procedure is illustrated in Figs. 12-1 through 12-11.

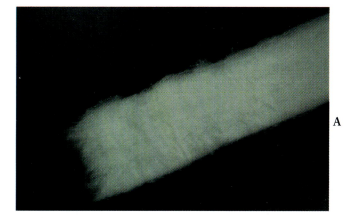

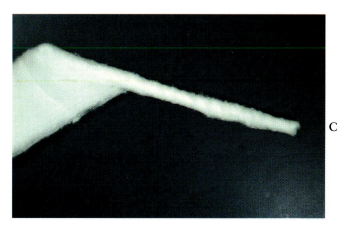

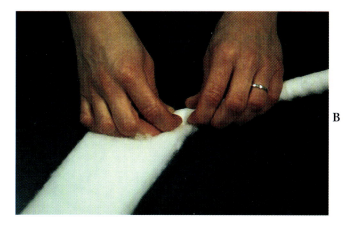

Fig. 12-1. A flat piece of cotton wool is twisted into a firm, cotton-wool roll with a diameter of ± 2 cm. Over the tibia and around the knee, we use rolls of decreased firmness to prevent the formation of bullae or damage to saphenous or peroneal nerves.

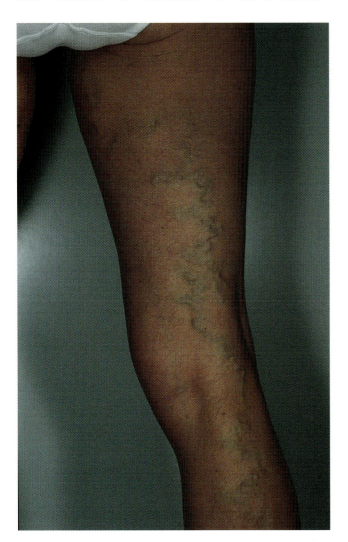

Fig. 12-2.   Strongly wound insufficient posterolateral branch.

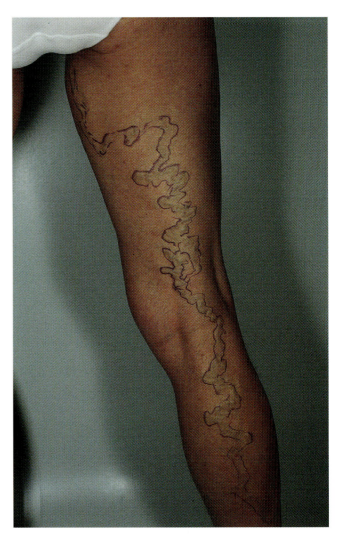

Fig. 12-3.   The course of the varicose veins is carefully marked when the patient is standing.

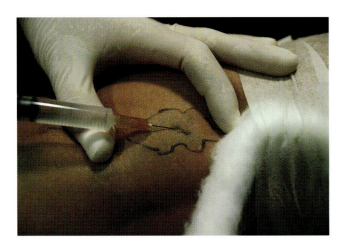

Fig. 12-4.   The injections are given when the patient is in the supine position. If necessary, we use the venous Doppler ultrasound to determine the exact location of an incompetent perforating vein or varicose vein that is clinically apparent in this position. The distance between injections is ± 5 cm. Approximately 0.25 cc. of sclerosing fluid is injected in each site. All varicose veins are treated at one time, provided that the total dose of sclerosant does not exceed maximal recommended amounts.

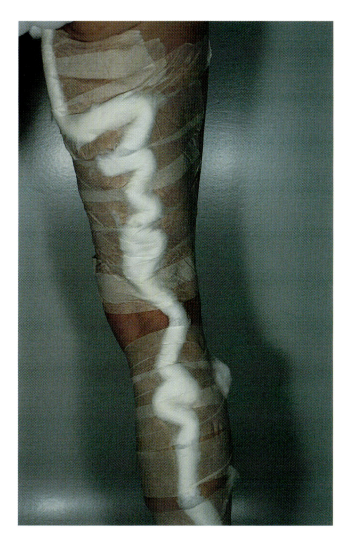

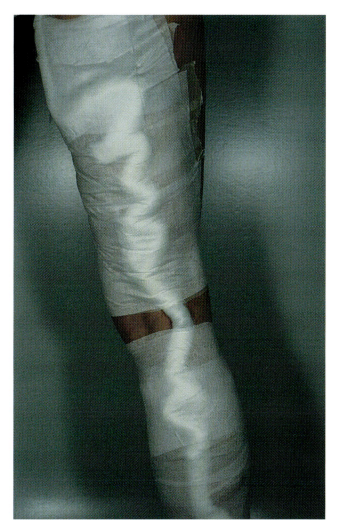

Fig. 12-5. The cotton-wool rolls follow the course of the varicose vein closely. We use fixation material on paper-base to prevent the formation of bullae on the edges (LeukoporR, 5 cm wide).

Fig. 12-6. For extra fixation we use broad, nonelastic fixation material (FixomullR stretch). The cotton-wool rolls submerge a bit in subcutaneous fat. We do not use fixation material in the hollow of the knee, so the function of the knee joint is not hampered.

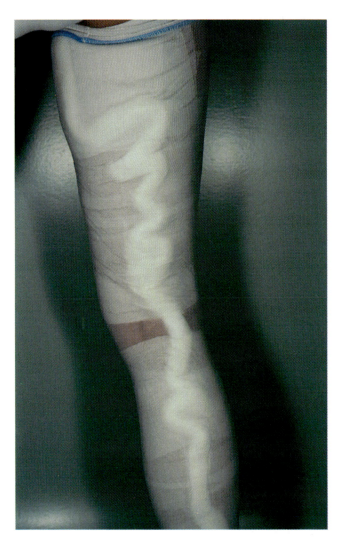

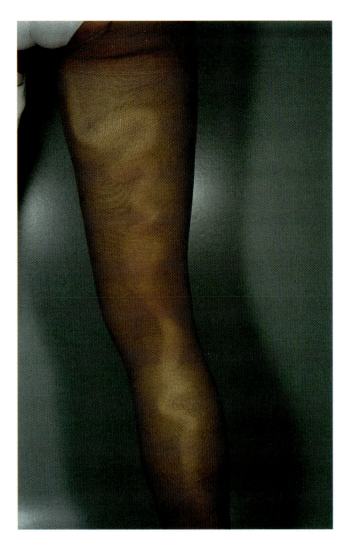

Fig. 12-7.   Class I stocking (ankle pressure ± 12 mmHg) for night and day.

Fig. 12-8.   Class II stocking (ankle pressure ± 30 mmHg) for the day.

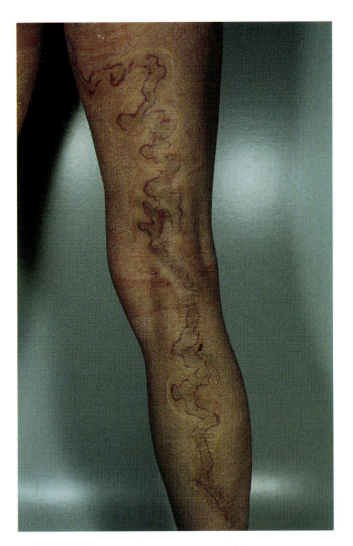

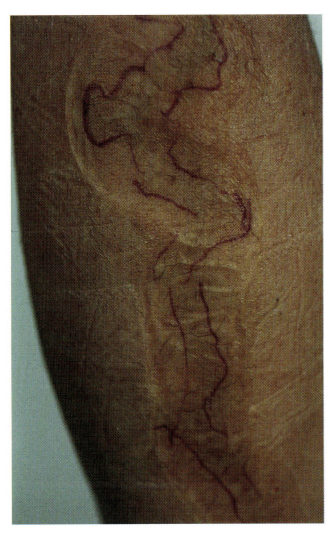

Fig. 12-9.   Checkup after one or two weeks. The impression in the skin is clearly visible after the removal of the pelottes. Depending on the amount of reflux before the treatment and the size of the treated varicose vein, new cotton-wool rolls are applied for one or two weeks or the patient only wears the class II stocking for one until four weeks.

Fig. 12-10.   Detail of the impression after the removal of the pelottes.

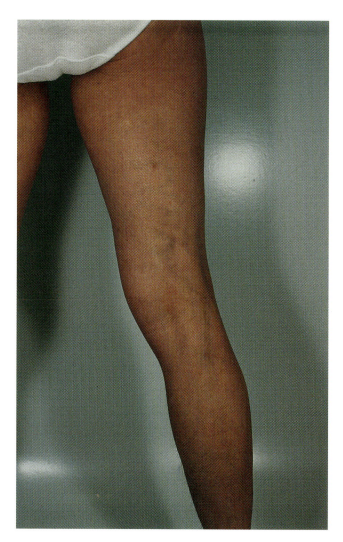

Fig. 12-11.   Situation after two months.

■ REFERENCES

1. Neumann HAM, Tazelaar DJ: Compression therapy. In Bergan JJ, Goldman MP, editors: Varicose veins and telangiectasias, diagnosis and treatment, St Louis, 1993, Quality Medical Publishing Inc.

2. Partsch H: Compression therapy of the legs, J Dermatol Surg Oncol 17:799-805, 1991.

3. Büller HR, Brandjes D, Ten Cate J: The post-thrombotic syndrome: prevention by elastic stockings, Beaune, France, 1993, International Union of Angiology.

4. Veraart JCJM, Verhaegh MEJM, Neumann HAM, Hulsmans RFHJ, Arends JW: Adhesion molecule expression in venous leg ulcers, VASA 22:213-218, 1993.

5. Fegan WG: Continuous compression technique of injecting varicose veins, The Lancet II:109-112, 1963.

6. Wallois P: Technique de la sclérose, Tournay R et al.: La sclérose des varices 189-199, Paris, 1980, Expansion Scientifique Française.

7. Stöberl CH, Gabler S, Partsch H: Indikations gerechte Bestrumpfung - Messung der venösen Pumpfunktion, Vasa 18:35-39, 1989.

8. Cleef JF van: Valves in varicose veins and external compression studied by angioscopy, Phlebology 8:116-119, 1993.

9. Fentem PH, Goddard M, Gooden BA et al.: Control of distention of varicose veins achieved by leg bandages, as used after injection sclerotherapy, Brit Med J 2:725-727, 1976.

10. Stemmer R: Konzentrische und exzentrische Kompression, Phlebologie und Proktologie 13:53-57, 1984.

11. Sarin S, Scurr JH, Coleridge Smith PD: Mechanism of action of external compression on venous function, Brit J Surg 79:499-502, 1992.

12. Raj TB, Goddard M, Makin GS: How long do compression bandages maintain their pressure during ambulatory treatment of varicose veins? Brit J Surg 67:122-124, 1980.

13. Bath AJ, Wickremesinghe SS, Gannon ME et al.: Randomised trial of bandaging after sclerotherapy for varicose veins, Brit Med J 1:423, 1980.

14. Fraser IA, Perry EP, Hatton M et al.: Prolonged bandaging is not required following sclerotherapy of varicose veins, Brit J Surg 72:488-490, 1985.

15. Wenner L: Gedanken über die Unterschiede bewährter Sklerotherapie-Methoden, Vasa 10:74-78, 1981.

16. Neumann HAM, Boersma IH: Light reflection rheography: a non-invasive diagnostic tool for screening for venous disease, J Dermatol Surg Oncol 18:425-430, 1992.

13

COMBINED TREATMENT, FLUSH LIGATION, AND COMPRESSION SCLEROTHERAPY FOR LARGE VARICOSE VEINS AND PERFORATORS

Joseph G. Sladen

Large varicose veins have been treated by intravenous injection for many years. During the 1940s many limbs were treated by high ligation and retrograde injection of sodium morrhuate into the long saphenous vein. This was fraught with complications including acute deep phlebitis. Sigg[1] introduced the addition of compression to sclerotherapy for large veins and perforator sites in 1952, and Fegan[2] popularized this in the English literature in the 1960s. A random trial comparing surgery with compression sclerotherapy published in 1974 by Hobbs[3] demonstrated that compression sclerotherapy controlled perforators effectively. The procedure described in this chapter is an "empty vein technique" used by all of the previously noted practitioners.[4] We added saphenofemoral "flush ligation" to our treatment 12 years ago because of poor results in the thigh using compression sclerotherapy alone in the presence of saphenofemoral reflux.[5,6]

◼ CLINICAL EXAMINATION

The examination aims at a specific anatomical diagnosis, for example, left saphenofemoral reflux or calf perforators (see Table 13-1).

◼ MANAGEMENT BEFORE INTERVENTION

The Pressure-Gradient Stocking

The pressure-gradient stocking is an integral part of treatment.[8] It serves as a therapeutic trial to confirm the diagnosis of venous insufficiency. A "sponge pump" (see following) is added if symptoms are severe, particularly if there is dermatitis, induration, or ulceration (Fig. 13-4). If complaints do not improve with pressure on follow-up examination, there is unrecognized arterial insufficiency or inadequate deep-venous collateral circulation or the diagnosis is in doubt.

If the calf portion of the stocking is too tight, the stocking acts like a tourniquet and exacerbates the symptoms with venous disease. Stretch the upper two inches of most stockings prior to use to achieve a comfortable fit. Apply the stocking by turning it inside out and then inverting the foot portion to the heel. The remaining stocking is everted over the foot and up the leg. The stocking should slip off the thumbs during this part of the application rather than being stretched up the leg. Avoid piling up the layers of the stocking particularly at the heel. There should be room for one or two fingers above the stocking in the popliteal fossa with the knee bent. It is important for the patient to learn to do this as the stocking will be used for compression following surgery and over the bandage after compression sclerotherapy.

The Sponge Pump

The sponge pump is made from soft, ½-inch latex foam rubber measuring approximately 8 × 20 cm (Fig. 13-4). It must be rounded and bevelled so that the edges do not indent the tissue when applied. The sponge pump is placed on the medial perforator region of the calf over the pressure-gradient stocking and wrapped with a 4-inch elastic bandage to apply extra pressure in this area. The bandage is applied tightly with crisscrossing spiral wraps on the lower part of the sponge and with less pressure applied to the upper part of the sponge by spreading out the wrapping and easing the pressure. The sponge pump can be modified by adding extra thickness to apply pressure behind the medial malleolus if required.

Table 13-1   Outline of Clinical Examination

1. Stand 10 minutes.	*Standing loads the venous system and usually brings out the patient's symptoms.*
2. Insonate with the Doppler about 8 cm below the inguinal ligament while compressing and releasing the long saphenous vein on the medial aspect of the thigh (Fig. 13-1). Note reflux when the hand is released over the saphenous and enhancement with a Valsalva's maneuver.	*Patient blows against a hand pressed against the mouth.*
3. Identify short saphenous reflux posteriorly.	*The Doppler is also useful in examining the short saphenous system, but it is more difficult to be anatomically specific about reflux in the popliteal fossa because of the adjacent deep venous system. A contrast varicogram is very helpful in identifying the level of the short saphenous popliteal vein junction if the vein is incompetent.[7]*
4. Identify thigh perforators by occluding the saphenous vein with a finger above while insonating with the Doppler below.	
5. Identify control and entry points by manually stripping the veins proximally, then controlling the column of blood with the other hand. Blood suddenly fills the vein as the controlling hand moves up the leg past a control point or an incompetent perforator.	*Pressure applied at the control point above a nest of varicosities will prolong the filling time of the varicosities.*
6. Examine the anatomic perforator sites on the medial and posterior calf and thigh with the thumb, searching for tenderness and milking away the edema with repetitive pressure (Fig. 13-2).	*Frequently, a high-pressure perforator that has not been obvious emerges from the surrounding edema. The most important injection sites for compression sclerotherapy are fed by perforators or control points. They are often warm or tender.*
7. Use a venous form and diagram to record the patient's complaints and findings during examination (Fig. 13-3). Record the specific diagnosis.	*The form saves time and is very helpful when the patient returns for compression sclerotherapy.*

Patient Exercise

The patient is directed to walk two miles a day to ensure adequate deep-venous outflow. Patients who are unable to walk because of arthritis or cardiac problems are taught to exercise their calves against resistance. A bellows type of air-mattress foot pump works well for this purpose. If there is difficulty tolerating the stocking or the sponge pump, do not proceed with intervention, but persist in conservative management.

■ **FLUSH LIGATION**

If the patient has saphenofemoral reflux (60% of new patients with large varicosities), flush ligation of the origin of the saphenous vein is indicated.[4,8,9] The surgery is done on an outpatient basis under local anesthesia. The area is explored through a 5 cm incision on the groin crease over the saphenofemoral junction. All branches are carefully ligated with care taken not to miss collateral bypassing veins, which can cause recurrences.[10] The saphenous vein is divided. Large thigh perforators are probably best ligated at the time of flush ligation because they tend to recur after compression sclerotherapy alone. Large thigh varices are easily injected at the time of flush ligation. In this instance the patient is treated while supine on the operating table, and as many as six sites are injected. A folded abdominal dressing pad may be used if sponge is not available. A course of antiinflammatory medication and mild analgesic for one week reduces postoperative discom-

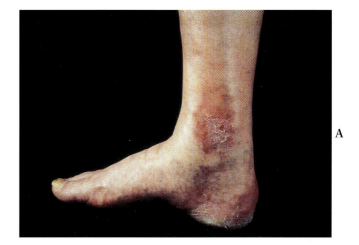

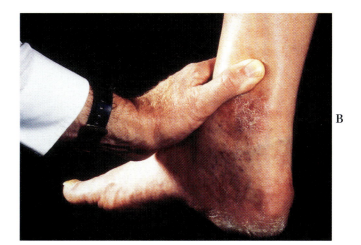

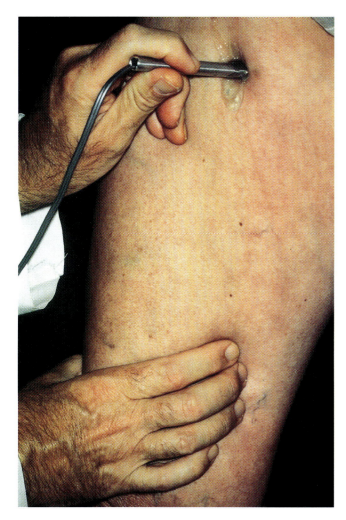

Fig. 13-1. Greater saphenous vein reflux is obtained by insonating the termination of the vein as shown here and compressing the distal pool.

fort. The patient should take three or four walks a day for a total of one mile. Most patients are ready to return to work three to four days after surgery.

■ COMPRESSION SCLEROTHERAPY

The patient must understand the basic principles of venous disease and learn to master the pressure-gradient stocking, which is an integral part of the treatment, before compression sclerotherapy. Therefore, compression sclerotherapy is never performed on the initial visit.

Injection tray

- Prefilled 3 ml syringes, 25 g needles
- 0.5 ml 1% and 3% sodium tetradecyl sulphate coded with tape

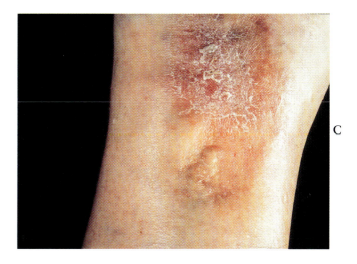

Fig. 13-2. **A** shows the severe cutaneous changes of chronic venous insufficiency. **B,** Firm pressure by the examining fingers or thumb will displace edema fluid and ease identification of perforating veins. **C,** After the edema is compressed, the perforating vein may be seen as a protuberant, saccular bulge, as shown.

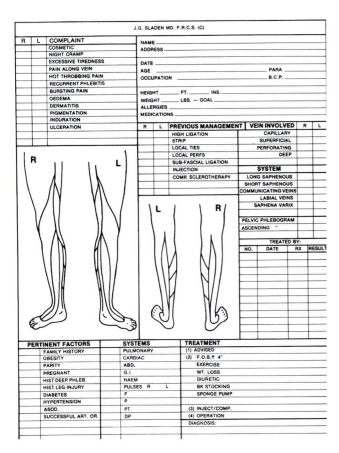

Fig. 13-3. Each physician will develop his or her own record form, but the one that has stood the test of time in our office is illustrated.

- Precut ½-inch tape, 8 cm lengths
- Cotton fluffs
- Crepe bandages
- Sponge
- Adhesive elastic bandage (Elastoplast)
- Scissors
- Porous plastic tape (micropore)

Other

- Foot stool (patient)
- Sitting stool (physician)
- Carpeting under examining table

An organized injection tray is mandatory if this procedure is to be accomplished expediently (Fig. 13-5). The suggested syringe and needle size provide good tactile feedback while the physician is injecting. A layer of carpeting under each end of the examining table allows the table to slide easily over a smooth floor.

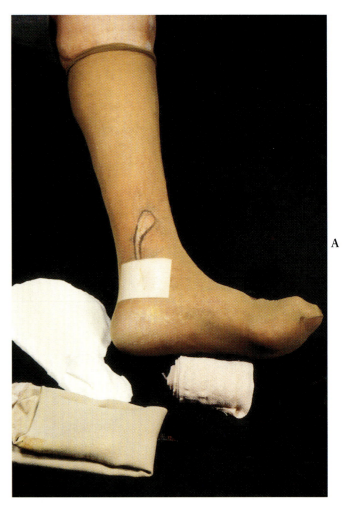

A

Fig. 13-4. The sponge pump shown has proved to be exceptionally useful in conservative treatment of the severe lipodermatosclerotic changes of chronic venous insufficiency. In **A** the sponge is seen adjacent to the treated ulcer and perforating vein.
—*Continued.*

■ TECHNIQUE

Table 13-2 outlines the technique to be followed.

■ FOLLOW-UP VISIT

The procedure for the follow-up examination is outlined in Table 13-3.

■ DIFFICULT AREAS

Compression sclerotherapy is most effective, and most easily performed, in the calf. However, it is often necessary to inject the thigh, ankle, or foot. A few helpful hints are offered here.

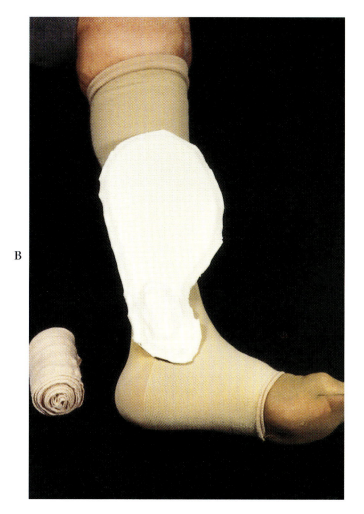

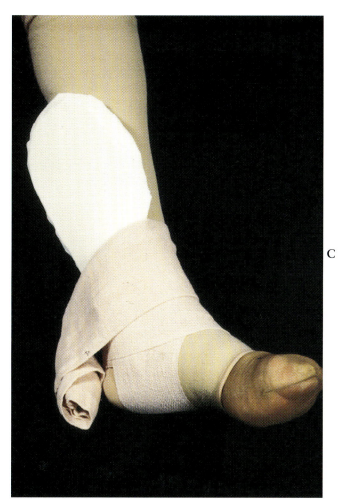

B

C

Fig. 13-4, cont'd. In **B** the foam rubber tailored to fit the ankle and leg has been applied, and in **C** elastic bandage is shown being applied to the ankle and the external sponge pump.

Thigh

Short-term and long-term results depend on control of saphenofemoral incompetency.[4,5,9] Ligation of a large perforator is an easy addition to flush ligation under local anesthesia.

Wrapping should be continued across the knee to avoid pooling in this area. Use half of a dressing pad in the popliteal fossa to prevent bunching of the bandage (Fig. 13-9, *A*). Maintaining compression over thigh varicosities can be very difficult. It can be useful to apply tincture of benzoin to the skin at the upper end of the bandage and overlap the adhesive elastic bandage onto the skin for a border of about 2 cm, warning the patient of the danger of skin reaction. The bandage

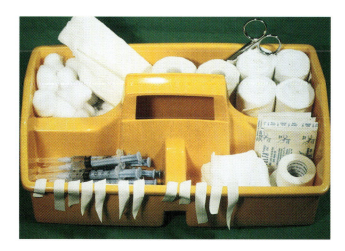

Fig. 13-5. An organized injection tray considerably speeds the treatment of patients by sclerotherapy. The tray used in our office is shown with its precut strips of tape, the filled syringes, cottonballs, and other necessary equipment.

on the thigh holds the sponge in place, but compression is maintained by rewrapping a 6-inch elastic bandage over the crepe bandage (Fig. 13-9, A). This usually needs to be done every two or three days and in some cases daily.[8] When the crepe bandage and sponge compression slip, the thigh bandage must be rewrapped so that the sponge again follows the course of the sclerosed vein. Most patients can manage this themselves, but some return for rewrapping.

Limbs that have been injected in the thigh frequently require aspiration of intravascular thrombus after compression sclerotherapy.

Ankle

Bandages that incorporate the ankle can cause blisters and sometimes ulceration over the Achilles tendon because of pressure and friction. Friction can be reduced by covering the area with a nonstick dressing (Telfa) or a thin plastic wrap, before bandaging. Smaller cotton fluffs are used on the foot, supplemented with a piece of half-inch foam, custom fitted, and bevelled to cover the injection sites. This reduces the bulk so that a shoe can be worn.

■ COMPLICATIONS

Warn the patient about superficial phlebitis (usually localized), pigmentation, and injection ulcers. Saphenous neuritis is rare. Itchiness following injection is a warning of developing sensitivity. Anaphylactic reaction is extremely rare (1 in 10,000). Aspiration of thrombus immediately reduces pain and reduces pigmentation. Pigmentation improves over the first year, but the residual staining may be permanent. It compares favorably with the appearance of a large vein prior to treatment.

Ulceration occurs in 3% of limbs after compression sclerotherapy of large veins (Fig. 13-10, A). The ulcers are not painful and are easily managed with a small, dry dressing under a pressure-gradient stocking. The scar (Fig. 13-10, B) can be excised through a very acceptable incision.

■ RECURRENCES

Recurrences, particularly at the site of high-pressure perforators are not uncommon (20% at four years), but can easily be retreated with compression

---

Table 13-2   Technique

Patient stands for 10 minutes.	*Standing makes the veins more turgid, which facilitates needle placement within the vein lumen. Some patients are prone to vasovagal syncope and can be treated sitting or on a tilt table if the veins are palpable in that position.*
Mark injection sites.	
Introduce the needle into the vein obliquely so that there is good tissue friction along the needle (Fig. 13-6).	*A flash of blood into the needle hub indicates that the needle is in the vein lumen. We usually do not inject the saphenous trunk.*
Use 3% in the large, deep veins and 1% in the smaller and more superficial veins.	*The incidence of injection ulcer is lower with 1% concentration, but 3% is more effective, particularly over a perforator.*
Secure the syringe to the leg with ½-inch tape.	
When all the needles have been placed, move the examining table to the patient and help the patient to the supine position. Support the limb in transit. Elevate the leg with the foot rested on the physician's shoulder.	*Elevation empties the veins. The veins are actually injected with the limb against the physician's chest or suspended in a sling.*
Starting distally, inject the sclerosant slowly from each syringe, trapping it by digital pressure applied through a cotton fluff placed about 6 cc proximal to the injection site.	*Warn the patient to report severe stinging (like a "bee sting"). This usually means that the sclerosant has extravasated, and the injection is stopped. Infiltration of 1% lidocaine solution controls the pain and may reduce the incidence of injection ulceration in this situation.*
As the needles are removed, control leakage of sclerosant by placing pressure over the needle hole in the vein with a cotton fluff, slightly proximal to the skin puncture site. If there are many injection sites on the leg, leave the syringes in place, removing them as the leg is wrapped.	*Often it is easier to inject and wrap the lower half of the leg and then proceed to the upper half. It may be better tolerated by some patients to break this into two sessions of compression sclerotherapy, injecting the calf prior to the thigh. Similarly, varicosities of the foot are more easily managed after treating the calf.*

—Continued.

Table 13-2 Technique —cont'd.

Apply precut tapered 1 inch latex sponge rubber along the course of the vein, which can be seen by the outline of the cotton fluffs through the crepe bandage. Compress the sponge with another layer of wrapping.	*Pressure can be increased by collapsing the sponge with finger pressure prior to wrapping over perforator sites. In a lean limb, tension must be reduced slightly over the anterior border of the tibia or the bandage may cause burning or blistering. In a large leg, compressing the sponge with a thumb as it is being wrapped produces more pressure locally over the course of the vein. The wrap must be applied smoothly.[11]*
Apply a third wrap, (usually a second crepe bandage), in random fashion to support, but not compress the whole area.	*This results in almost a castlike firmness without excessive pressure.*
Add adhesive elastic bandages at the top and bottom of the bandage for stability, avoiding contact with the skin.	
Cover the bandage with an old nylon stocking. Evert the foot of the pressure-gradient stocking and slide it over the nylon.	*Bandages are covered with an old nylon stocking, which is used both day and night to protect the bandage and to aid in applying the pressure-gradient stocking.*
Record injection and suspected extravasation sites on the vein form.	
Apply a nylon stocking over the bandage day and night.	*The nylon stocking is used to protect the bandage both day and night.*
Walk two miles a day, divided in three or four sessions.	*Warn the patient that the foot may be cyanotic and congested when dependent, but that this is controlled by the pressure-gradient stocking and walking. Patients who are unable to walk use an air-mattress foot pump or treadle.*
Ease pressure at ankle and foot if necessary by loosening the outer wrap of the bandage and cutting the lower edge.	*Instruct patients to cut the lower edge of the bandage if the foot swells excessively or if the bandage cuts in. Accomplish this by cutting approximately one third of the width of the bandage in successive layers at the 4, 8, and 12 o'clock positions. Avoid exposing the skin; it only moves the problem proximally. Reapply the adhesive elastic bandage to produce a neat bandage with tapered pressure.*
Apply additional pressure over tender areas.	*Apply pressure with a sanitary napkin or similar pad over any area of tenderness and wrap the area with an elastic bandage.*
Remove the bandage in three weeks.	*The patient removes the bandages in three weeks if large high-pressure veins were treated or in ten days if smaller lower-pressure veins were injected. A handout guides the patient through this period. Examine the patient three or four days after the bandage is removed. There should be no interruption in the patient's work schedule unless there is a great deal of standing or kneeling in the patient's work place.*

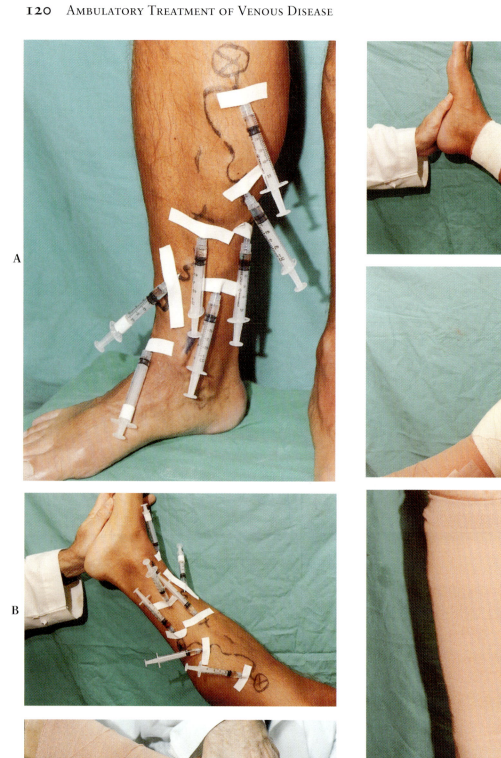

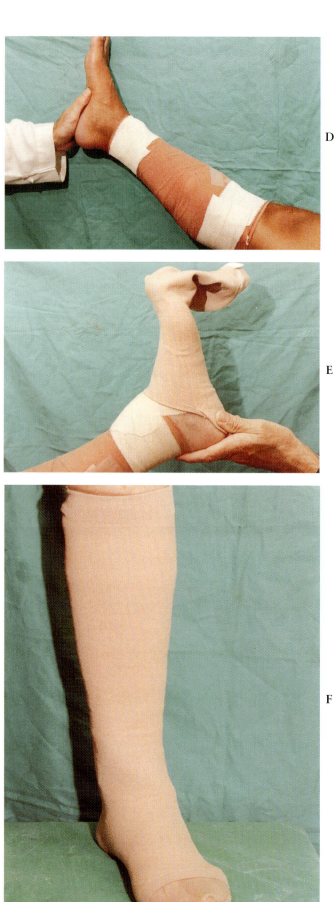

sclerotherapy.[12] Large thigh recurrences, or recurrences in the groin from previous inadequate flush ligation, are often best treated with surgery. A preoperative varicogram can be helpful in defining the problem.[13]

VENOUS ULCERATION

Venous ulceration represents the severe end of the venous-disease spectrum. After controlling and healing a venous ulcer, combined treatment is useful in maintaining control.

Venous ulcers are healed by applying pressure directly over the ulcer and feeding perforator sites. Patients should be instructed that "pressure heals." The ulcers are usually not painful; if they are, there is likely to be either a significant infective component or an ischemic element (arterial occlusive disease or hypertension).

Most patients can be treated on an ambulatory basis, and this should be a goal of treatment.

Treatment of Venous Ulcers

The ulcer should be covered with a gauze dressing, changed daily. This should be backed with a portion of abdominal dressing, held in place with a nylon stocking. This dressing should be covered with a pressure-gradient stocking. A "sponge pump" is applied over the stocking; the rubber is sculpted to fit behind the malleolus where necessary and held in place with an elastic bandage to apply pressure directly over the ulcer and perforator sites.

Patients are instructed to walk two miles per day. Healing occurs at approximately 1 cm per month. A nonstick (Telfa) pad is substituted for the gauze, and the abdominal pad is eliminated when the ulcer is dry.

Combined treatment is effective in maintaining control of healed ulcers. Injection is delayed until it can be done through normal or near-normal subcutaneous tissue. These patients should continue to wear a pressure-gradient stocking permanently. Compliance has been good in our experience, with ulcer recurrence of 3% at four years, confirming the work of others.[14]

Fig. 13-6. (**Facing Page**) Injections are performed with the limb dependent and the patient in the standing position to fill the veins to be treated. In **A** we see that the injection sites have been marked, and the needle has been placed within the lumen of each vein to be injected. The needles are taped into place, and the syringes are now dependent. In **B** the leg is elevated to empty the veins, and the limb is held in an elevated position by the patient's pressing the foot against the physician's chest or suspended by the nursing assistant. In **C**, starting distally, the injection is placed slowly from each syringe. The sclerosant is concentrated in the injection site by trapping it between the fingers of the operator's left hand as shown here. **D**, Cotton fluff is placed over each needle-puncture hole. Precut sponge rubber can be placed along the course of the veins, and the leg carefully wrapped as indicated in the text. An old nylon stocking covers the preliminary wrap so that the pressure-gradient stocking can be applied as shown in **E**. The completed bandaging and stocking application is shown in **E**. Instructions are then given as indicated in the text regarding further care.

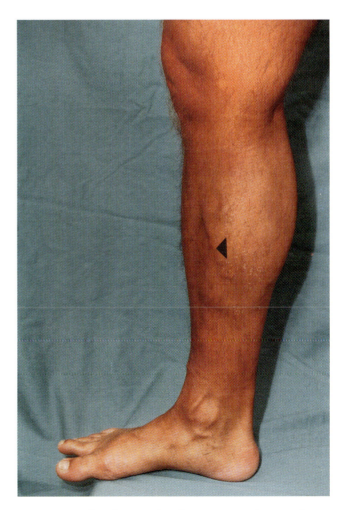

Fig. 13-7. After three weeks of compression therapy, the patient returns to the office and stands as shown here. Residual varicosities are searched for, and as indicated by the arrow, thrombus or entrapped blood is also noted.

Table 13-3   Follow-up Visit

Stand briefly (Fig. 13-7).	*Examine the patient in the standing or sitting position for residual varicosities and thrombus (arrow) and thrombus.*
Inject the remaining varicose veins if necessary.	*Manage residual veins with repeat compression sclerotherapy.*
Aspirate intravenous thrombus and apply pressure for four days (Fig. 13-8).	*Aspirate intravenous thrombus if more than 3 mm in diameter with a 18 g needle and syringe or express after opening the skin with a #11 scalpel blade.*
Continue stocking at least three weeks.	*Continue the pressure-gradient stocking permanently if the patient suffers from deep-venous insufficiency.*
Add pressure to tender areas.	*Place a pad under the pressure-gradient stocking or place the pad on top of the pressure-gradient stocking and wrap with tensor.*

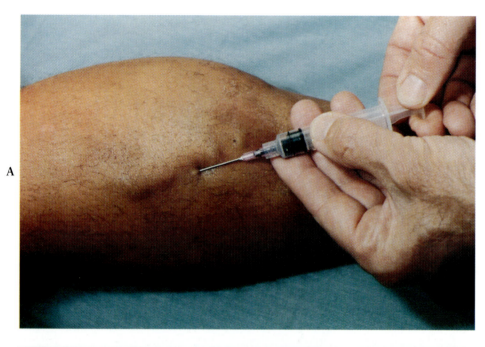

A

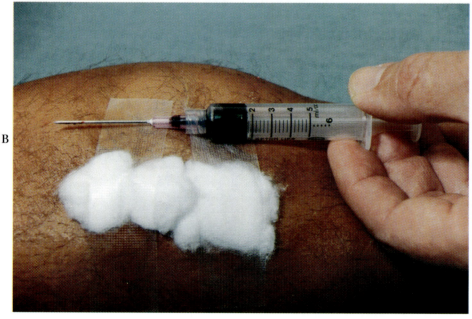

B

Fig. 13-8.   The entrapped blood may be treated as shown here. A #18 needle is inserted into the coagulum as shown in **A**, and aspiration completed as shown in **B**. Alternatively, a #11 blade can be used to evacuate the entrapped blood. A pressure dressing is applied for four days.

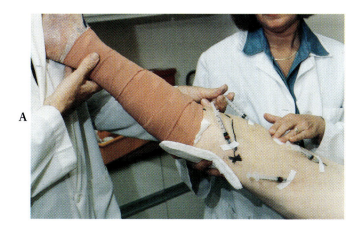
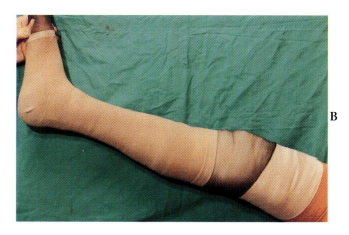

Fig. 13-9.   Compression after sclerotherapy in thigh veins may be difficult. As shown in **A**, the popliteal fossa is protected from bunching of the bandage, and, as shown in **B**, a pressure bandage is applied to give continuity between the distal stocking and the proximal compression bandage. The thigh elastic bandage may need to be rewrapped to keep continuous compression in place.

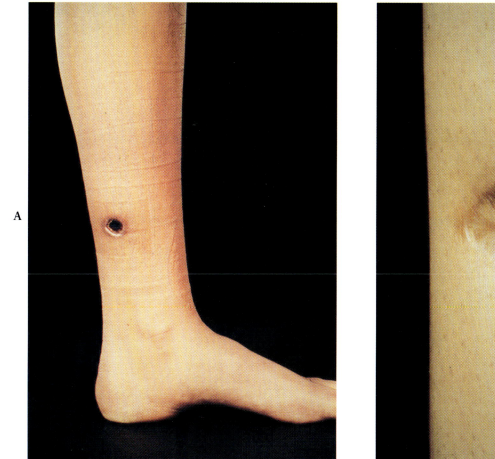
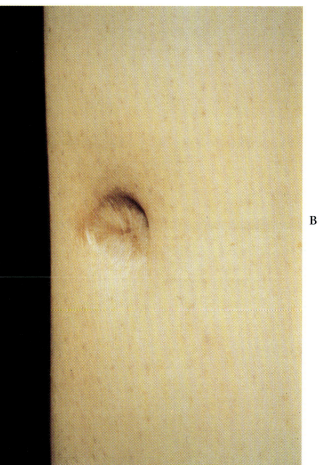

Fig. 13-10.   A complication of compression sclerotherapy is skin ulceration. The ulcers are circular and punched out sharply, but quite deep as shown here in **A**. They are best managed by a dry dressing and pressure-gradient stocking, and the resultant scar as shown in **B** can be excised to provide an acceptable cosmetic result.

■ SUMMARY

Large varicosities and perforator disease are effectively managed through "combined" treatment. Treatment can be repeated easily when necessary. This treatment is not surgery free, is not a cure, and rarely produces a "Hollywood leg." It is particularly suited to the elderly, obese, and high-risk patient with symptomatic disease.

■ REFERENCES

1. Sigg K: The treatment of varicosities and accompanying complications, Angiology 3:355-379, 1952.

2. Fegan WB: Continuous compression technique of injecting varicose veins, Lancet 3:109-112, 1963.

3. Hobbs JT: Surgery and sclerotherapy in the treatment of varicose veins: a random trial, Arch Surg 109:793-796, 1974.

4. Sladen JG: Flush ligation and compression sclerotherapy in the control of venous disease, Am J Surg 152:535-538, 1986.

5. McCaffery J: An approach to the treatment of varicose veins, Med J Aust 1:1379, 1969.

6. Sladen JG: Compression sclerotherapy: preparation, technique, complications, and results, Am J Surg 146:228-232, 1983.

7. Hobbs JT: Perioperative venography to ensure accurate sapheno-popliteal vein ligation, Br Med J 2:1578-1580, 1980.

8. Raj TB, Goddard M, Makin GS: How long do compression bandages maintain their pressure during ambulatory treatment of varicose veins? Br J Surg 67:122-124, 1980.

9. Burnand JG, O'Donnell TF, Thomas ML, Browse NL. The relative importance of incompetent communicating veins in the production of varicose veins and venous ulcers, Surgery 82:9-14, 1977.

10. Hobbs JT: Operations for varicose veins. In De Weese JA, editor: Rob and Smith's Operative Surgery, Vascular Surgery, 4th ed. St Louis, 1985, Mosby and London, 1985, Butterworths, p 278.

11. Fegan WG: The art of bandaging the lower limb. Br J Hospital Medicine :697-698, 1971.

12. Sladen JG: Complicated deep venous insufficiency: conservative management, Canadian J Surg 29:No 1, 17-18,1986.

13. Thomas ML, Bowles JN: Incompetent perforating veins: comparison of varicography and ascending phlebography, Radiology 154:619-623, 1985.

14. Henry MEF, Fegan WG, Pegum JM: Five-year survey of the treatment of varicose ulcers, Br Med J 2:493-494, 1971.

14

MACROSCLEROTHERAPY OF VENOUS JUNCTIONS

Pauline Raymond-Martimbeau

In sclerotherapy of varicose vein disease, the first goal is to eliminate the highest point of reflux, thereby decreasing the distal venous pressure. The injection sequence then proceeds downward until all incompetent sites have been treated.[1-3] In some cases, eradicating the highest point of reflux will automatically eliminate distal varicosities without further treatment. In all cases, such eradication is crucial for preventing post-sclerotherapeutic complications, vein recanalization, and neovascularization.

VENOUS JUNCTIONAL ANATOMY

Saphenofemoral Junction

In most individuals (91.4%),[4,5] the greater (long) saphenous vein (Fig. 14-1) and the common femoral vein join at Scarpa's triangle, at the groin level, to form the saphenofemoral junction (Fig. 14-2). The greater saphenous vein has a single, uninterrupted trunk in 84.3% of cases, a double trunk in 12.2%, and a triple trunk in 3.5%.[6,7]

Saphenopopliteal Junction

In 42.4% of cases, the lesser (short) saphenous vein terminates in the popliteal vein, at the popliteal crease, to form the saphenopopliteal junction (Fig. 14-3). Alternatively, this junction can occur above the popliteal crease (12.8% of cases) or below it (6.6%).[4] In 38.2% of patients, the lesser saphenous vein terminates in a vein other than the popliteal.[5] Nevertheless, this site is generally still referred to as the saphenopopliteal junction. In 10% to 20% of patients, the lesser saphenous vein is duplicated.[5]

In most cases (82.7%),[4] the greater and lesser saphenous veins are joined by anastomotic veins, the most important of which is Giacomini's vein (Fig. 14-4).

Because the saphenofemoral and saphenopopliteal junctions are particularly vulnerable to valvular malfunction, one of them often proves to be the highest point of reflux. In such cases, the initial sclerotherapeutic injection must eliminate backflow at the junction in question.

TREATMENT GOALS

During the past decade, protocols for sclerosing the venous junctions have become standardized,[7-11] and increasing experience with injection at these sites has yielded consistently satisfactory results. For skilled practitioners the success rate approaches 90% (Figs. 14-5 through 14-7).[12] Nevertheless, because the anatomy in these areas tends to be complex, such injection should be attempted only by experienced sclerotherapists. These individuals should be familiar with duplex monitoring techniques to allow adequate pretherapeutic assessment of venous topography and morphology. In selected cases, the sclerotherapeutic procedure itself may be performed with duplex ultrasonographic guidance.

Ideally, sclerotherapy should produce the following results, as documented by intravenous ultrasound.[7] Within 20 minutes of injection, the traumatized endothelium undergoes circumferential thickening (Fig. 14-8). This stage is followed by development of a thrombus-like formation, which adheres to the endothelium. After a variable interval, the lumen is obliterated, causing the vein to shrink in diameter. The vein then undergoes fibrosis (Fig. 14-9) and is ultimately reabsorbed. From a clinical standpoint, it should be indurated, but neither painful nor inflamed.

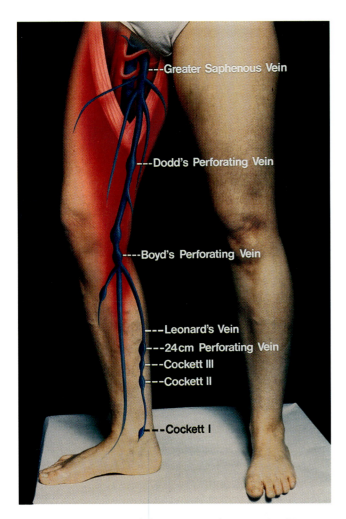

Fig. 14-1. Anatomy of the greater saphenous vein. (From Raymond-Martimbeau P: Color atlas of sclerotherapy for varicose and telangiectatic veins, Dallas, 1994, PRM Editions [in press]).

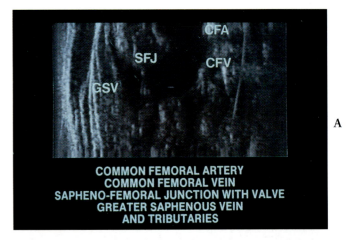

A

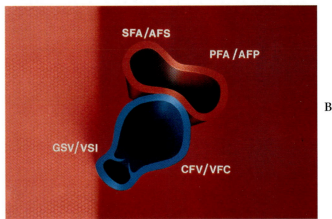

B

Fig. 14-2. **A,** Duplex ultrasonogram showing a transverse section of the saphenofemoral junction. The ostial valve is clearly visible. CFA = common femoral artery; CFV = common femoral vein; GSV = greater saphenous vein; SFJ = saphenofemoral junction. **B,** Diagrammatic cross-section of the saphenofemoral junction. CFV/VFC = common femoral vein; GSV/VSI = greater saphenous vein; PFA/AFP = profunda femoris artery; SFA/AFS = superficial femoral artery. (From Raymond-Martimbeau P: Color atlas of sclerotherapy for varicose and telangiectatic veins, Dallas, 1994, PRM Editions.

If this process is incomplete or otherwise unsuccessful, it will bypass the endothelium and, instead, affect the adventitia and surrounding tissue. These structures will undergo thickening, and the thrombus will form too early, failing to adhere to the nonreactive intima. Thickening of the adventitia and surrounding tissues will cause the venous diameter to expand. This process can result in an excessive inflammatory reaction, which can lead to cutaneous hyperpigmentation (Fig. 14-10). In such cases, the vein becomes indurated, inflamed, and painful. It may eventually recanalize or undergo neovascularization.

The following points apply only to straightforward cases, in which neither clinical examination, including palpation and percussion (Schwartz maneuver), nor ultrasonographic studies reveal any variant saphenous vein terminations or other anatomic irregularities.

■ TYPE AND DOSAGE OF SCLEROSANT

The classification of sclerosing agents has already been described elsewhere.[6] Injection of either venous junction necessitates a major sclerosant. Major agents used worldwide include iodine sodium iodide[13] (iodine USP or sodium iodide USP, in crystal form [Fisher Scientific Company, Fair Lawn, New Jersey]; Sclerodine [Omega Laboratories, Montreal]; Variglobin [Globopharm SA, Zurich]) and sodium tetradecyl sulfate (So-

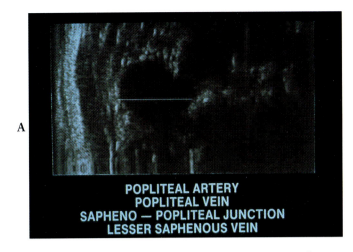

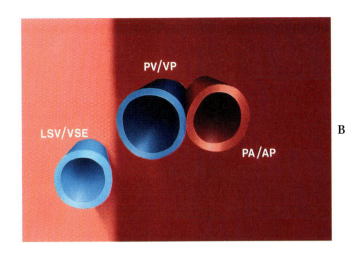

A   B

Fig. 14-3.   **A,** Duplex ultrasonogram showing a transverse section of the saphenopopliteal junction. The lesser saphenous vein terminates in the popliteal vein. **B,** Diagrammatic cross-section of the saphenopopliteal junction. LSV/VSE = lesser saphenous vein; PA/AP = popliteal artery; PV/VP = popliteal vein. (From Raymond-Martimbeau P: Color atlas of sclerotherapy for varicose and telangiectatic veins, Dallas, 1994, PRM Editions.)

tradecol [Wyeth, Philadelphia]); Thromboject [Omega Laboratories, Montreal]; Trombovar [Promedica, France]). Injection at these sites should not be attempted with an intermediate or a minor sclerosing agent. These solutions would not be strong enough to induce an immediate endothelial reaction, but would, instead, diffuse distally, increasing the risk of an excessive inflammatory reaction.

As a general rule, the initial dose for injecting the saphenofemoral junction is 2 ml of 3% iodine sodium iodide or 2 ml of 2% sodium tetradecyl sulfate. For the saphenopopliteal junction, the initial dose is generally

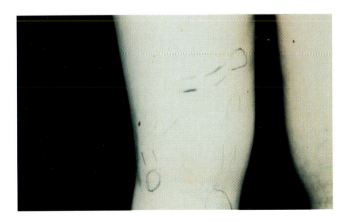

Fig. 14-4.   Incompetence of Giacomini's vein. (From Raymond-Martimbeau P: Color atlas of sclerotherapy for varicose and telangiectatic veins, Dallas, 1994, PRM Editions.)

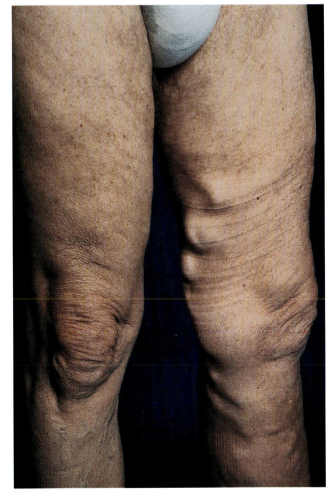

Fig. 14-5.   Incompetence of the saphenofemoral junction and perforating veins before sclerotherapy. (From Raymond-Martimbeau P: Color atlas of sclerotherapy for varicose and telangiectatic veins, Dallas, 1994, PRM Editions.)

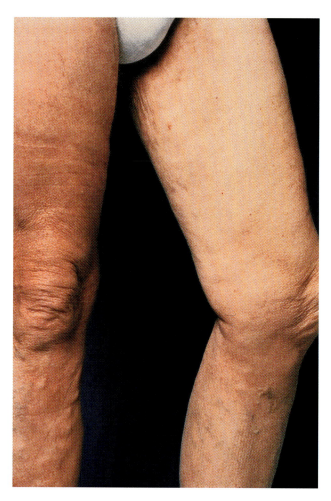

Fig. 14-6. Postsclerotherapeutic view of the structures shown in Fig. 14-5. (From Raymond-Martimbeau P: Color atlas of sclerotherapy for varicose and telangiectatic veins, Dallas, 1994, PRM Editions.)

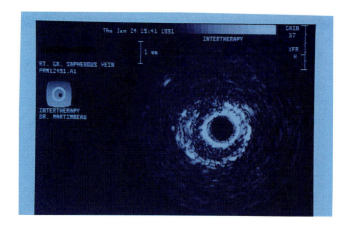

Fig. 14-8. Intravenous ultrasonogram showing a 360° cross-sectional image of the greater saphenous vein after sclerotherapy. Note the circumferential endothelial thickening. (From Raymond-Martimbeau P: Color atlas of sclerotherapy for varicose and telangiectatic veins, Dallas, 1994, PRM Editions.)

1 ml of either major sclerosant, in a concentration of 1%. If further treatment of these sites is necessary, the concentration should be increased by 1% at each subsequent session, while the volume remains the same. Because the target is highly specific, success depends upon immediate contact between the sclerosant and the endothelium. If an immediate endothelial reaction is not induced by a standard dose, adding more volume will be ineffective.

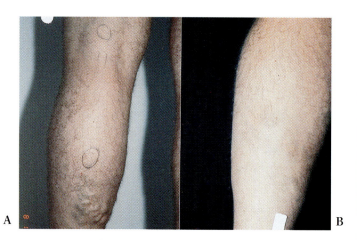

A   B

Fig. 14-7. Incompetence of the saphenopopliteal junction and of a perforating vein before **A** and after **B** sclerotherapy. (From Raymond-Martimbeau P: Color atlas of sclerotherapy for varicose and telangiectatic veins, Dallas, 1994, PRM Editions.)

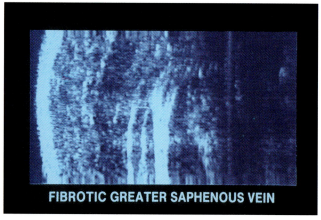

FIBROTIC GREATER SAPHENOUS VEIN

Fig. 14-9. Duplex ultrasonogram revealing a fibrotic reaction of the greater saphenous vein. (From Raymond-Martimbeau P: Role of sclerotherapy in greater saphenous vein incompetence. From Raymond-Martimbeau P: Color atlas of sclerotherapy for varicose and telangiectatic veins, Dallas, 1994, PRM Editions [in press].)

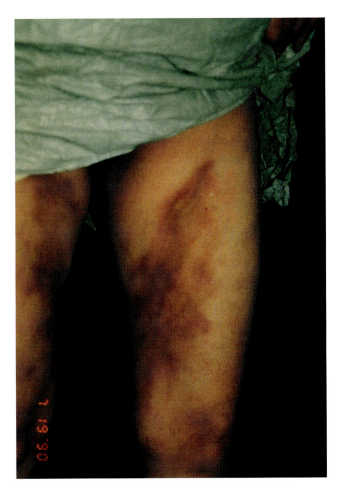

Fig. 14-10. Cutaneous hyperpigmentation seven years after injection of the greater saphenous vein with sodium tetradecyl sulfate. (From Raymond-Martimbeau P: Color atlas of sclerotherapy for varicose and telangiectatic veins, Dallas, 1994, PRM Editions.)

◼ TECHNIQUE

General Considerations

Eradicating reflux at a venous junction is usually accomplished with a single injection, given several centimeters below—rather than right at—the junction in question (Fig. 14-11).[12] This slightly indirect approach helps avoid inadvertent puncture of the deep-venous or arterial system. Multiple injections could induce distal occlusion, with residual permeability at the junction, thereby increasing venous pressure and possibly causing an inflammatory reaction, which could result in hyperpigmentation and recanalization.

It is important that the physician follow a logical treatment plan and not be tempted to skip steps. The protocol is the same for all veins, regardless of their size. One might assume that larger doses are needed for larger veins, but this is not true. In fact, injecting an excessive initial dose of a major sclerosant into a large vein can cause premature, nonadherent thrombus formation, with the risk of complications.

As in injecting other points of reflux, the physician should confirm the location and depth of the venous junction by means of percussion (Fig. 14-12). Once the skin has been cleansed with alcohol, the vein is entered briskly with a needle that is large enough to not accidentally enter a small artery and short enough to not enter the deep-venous system. A few drops of blood are withdrawn to verify proper needle positioning. Accidental penetration of an artery is heralded by pulsating, bright-red blood; if such flow is observed, immediate withdrawal of the needle is imperative. Injection should always be postponed until correct needle positioning is assured.

Once the physician is certain that it is safe to proceed, the sclerosant is administered as follows: The first half of the dose is given very slowly, and the needle position is again confirmed by means of aspiration; the rest of the dose is then given rapidly, and the needle is withdrawn swiftly, without letting any drops of sclerosant come in contact with the skin. Pain during the injection process may herald a serious complication, so the patient should speak up at once if any discomfort is felt. Likewise, any other unusual symptom should be reported immediately.

Saphenofemoral Junction

Sound protocols for the saphenofemoral junction have been described elsewhere[1,8-10,12] and are summarized in Tables 14-1 and 14-2.

Two patient positions (sitting and standing) have been described for injecting this site (Fig. 14-13):[12] When the *sitting position* is used, the patient's leg is abducted and rotated externally, and the knee is flexed.[1,8-10,12] The physician remains standing. With this approach, a disposable 3-ml syringe is used, with a disposable standard 25-gauge, ⅝-inch (1.6 cm) needle. The injection is given 5 to 9 cm below the junction.[14] Digital pressure is applied at the junction during the injection and for 1 minute afterward.[8-10,14]

When the *standing position* is used, the patient should be positioned on a surface large enough to allow slight spreading of the legs. The author prefers a specially designed 20 × 20-inch cube for this purpose (Fig. 14-14). For optimum stability, the patient's heels should be at the same level, and his or her weight should be placed on the leg to be injected. To facilitate exposure, this leg should be abducted and rotated

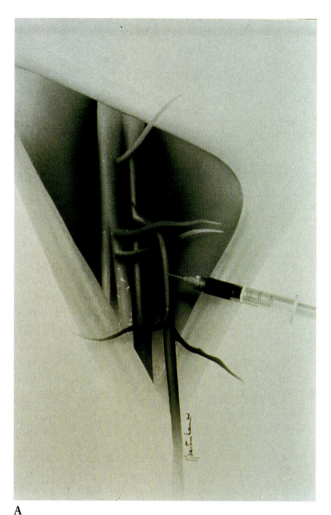

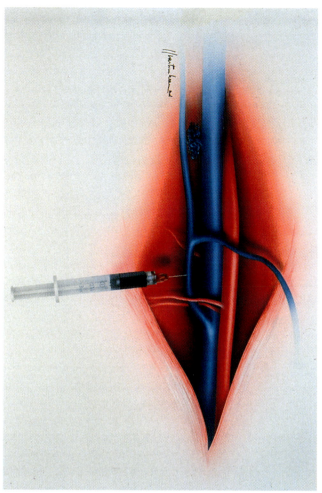

A   B

Fig. 14-11. Single injection, given several centimeters below the venous junction: **A,** sapheno-femoral junction; **B,** saphenopopliteal junction. (From Raymond-Martimbeau P: Role of sclerotherapy in greater saphenous vein incompetence. In Bergan JJ, Goldman MP, editors: Varicose veins and telangiectasias: diagnosis and treatment, St Louis, 1993, Quality Medical Publishing, pp 226–258.)

externally; the patient should look straight ahead and not lean on anything. The physician should be seated on an adjustable stool.

With this approach, it is sometimes advisable to use a disposable 25-gauge, ⅝-inch (1.6 cm) butterfly needle, with 12 inches (30 cm) of tubing.

The injection should be given 4 to 7 cm below the saphenofemoral junction. Digital compression should be exerted both at the junction and below the site of injection to sequester the venous trunk and allow maximal selective endothelial contact. (The author was the first to describe this sequestration technique, which greatly enhances the sclerosing process.[12]) Once the injection has been completed, distal compression is terminated, but pressure over the junction is maintained for an additional minute.

Saphenopopliteal Junction

The saphenopopliteal junction is injected with a 1-ml disposable syringe and a disposable 26-gauge, ½-inch (1.3 cm) needle.[7]

The patient may lie prone, kneel, or stand with the leg flexed. (The author prefers the latter position.) In all other respects, the procedure is similar to that described earlier (Fig. 14-15).

Other Sites of Disease

After reflux has been abolished at the venous junction, the entire involved saphenous vein should be treated, as clinically indicated, by injecting the next highest site of reflux with a major sclerosing agent. As the injection sequence proceeds downward, the concen-

Table 14-1 Schedule and Dosage of Iodine Sodium Iodide (Sclerodine)* Injections for Treating Greater Saphenous Vein Incompetence Secondary to Saphenofemoral Junctional (SFJ) Malfunction**

Visit	Dosage	Site
1	2 ml at 2% concentration	Below SFJ
2	2 ml at 3% concentration	Below SFJ
3	2 ml at 4% concentration	Below SFJ
	OR	
	2 ml at 3% concentration	Below SFJ
	1 ml at 3% concentration	Midthigh level
4	2 ml at 5% concentration	Below SFJ
	OR	
	2 ml at 3% concentration	Below SFJ
	1 ml at 3% concentration	Midthigh level
	1 ml at 2% concentration	Knee level

*Variglobin 2%, 4%, 8%, 12% is equivalent to Sclerodine solution 1%, 2%, 4%, 6%.
**Data from Raymond-Martimbeau P: Role of sclerotherapy in greater saphenous vein incompetence. In Bergan JJ, Goldman MP, editors: Varicose veins and telangiectasias: diagnosis and treatment, St Louis, 1993, Quality Medical Publishing, pp 226–258.

Table 14-2 Schedule and Dosage of Sodium Tetradecyl Sulfate Injections for Treating Greater Saphenous Vein Incompetence Secondary to Saphenofemoral Junctional (SFJ) Malfunction*

Visit	Dosage	Site
1	2 ml at 3% concentration	Below SFJ
2	2 ml at 4% concentration	Below SFJ
3	2 ml at 6% concentration	Below SFJ
4	2 ml at 6% concentration	Below SFJ
	1 ml at 3% concentration	Midthigh level
5	2 ml at 6% concentration	Below SFJ
	1 ml at 3% concentration	Midthigh level
	1 ml at 2% concentration	Knee level

*Data from Raymond-Martimbeau P: Two different techniques for sclerosing the incompetent saphenofemoral junction: a comparative study. J Dermatol Surg Oncol 16:626–631, 1990.

tration of sclerosant is decreased. As a rule, the dosages used are the following: 0.5 to 1.0 ml of a 3% sclerosant in the upper thigh; 0.5 to 1.0 ml of a 1.5% to 2% sclerosant in the lower thigh and upper leg; and 0.25 to 0.50 ml of a 1% sclerosant in the lower leg. In the author's opinion, concentrations of a major scle-

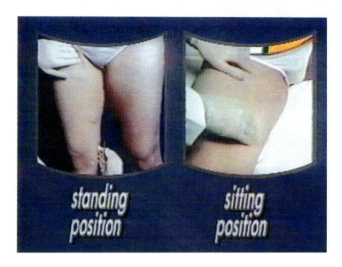

Fig. 14-12. Use of percussion to confirm the location and depth of the venous junction with the patient in **A,** the standing position and **B,** the sitting position. (From Raymond-Martimbeau P: Role of sclerotherapy in greater saphenous vein incompetence. In Bergan JJ, Goldman MP, editors: Varicose veins and telangiectasias: diagnosis and treatment, St Louis, 1993, Quality Medical Publishing, pp 226–258.)

rosant less than 1% in the saphenous systems will not induce an ideal permanent sclerotic reaction.

Once the involved vein has been treated, flow between the greater and lesser saphenous veins must be eliminated by treating the Giacomini and other anastomotic veins, thereby preventing disease recurrence. These veins are injected with 0.5 to 1.0 ml of a 1.5% to 2% major sclerosant.

■ POSTSCLEROTHERAPEUTIC CARE

After treatment of a saphenous junction, the patient should wear a noncircumferential selective compressive dressing for 48 hours. This regimen consists of numerous cotton balls, covered by several layers of 2-inch nonallergenic tape. For day wear, an elastic bandage or graduated compressive hosiery can be used (Fig. 14-16). To reduce venous congestion, patients are strongly advised to continue their normal activities and to pursue a low-impact postoperative exercise program.[1]

Careful follow-up study is an essential aspect of proper management. Because a single treatment is often insufficient to eradicate venous junctional reflux, additional injections can be undertaken at one- to three-week intervals (Tables 14-1 and 14-2). If three attempts have been made, using a maximal concentration of sclerosant at the junction, and if thickening of the endothelium has occurred, a composite technique using multiple injections may be necessary to induce the desired thrombus-like formation; in such a case, the

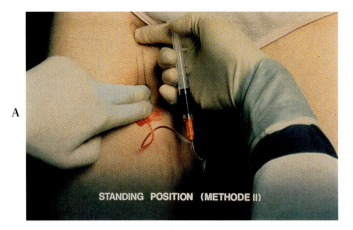

STANDING POSITION (METHODE II)

A

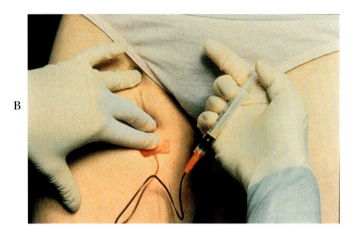

B

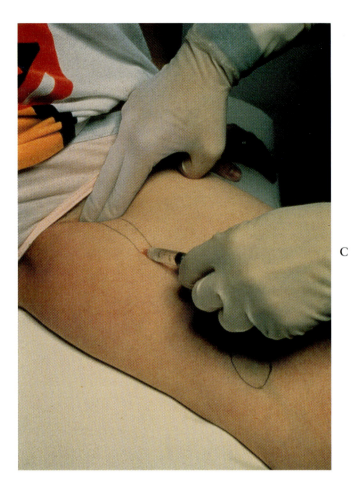

C

Fig. 14-13. **A,** Digital compression at the saphenofemoral junction and below the site of injection with the patient in the standing position. **B,** Variant of the standing position. **C,** Digital compression at the saphenofemoral junction only, with the patient in the sitting position. (From Raymond-Martimbeau P: Role of sclerotherapy in greater saphenous vein incompetence. In Bergan JJ, Goldman MP, editors: Varicose veins and telangiectasias: diagnosis and treatment, St Louis, 1993, Quality Medical Publishing, pp 226–258.)

effects of the multiple injections can reinforce each other (Fig. 14-17). If the outcome remains unsuccessful, the patient may benefit from surgery or a combined therapeutic approach.

◼ SUMMARY

In treating varicosities of the superficial venous system, injecting the saphenofemoral or saphenopopliteal junction is a valuable practice that appears well tolerated when clinically indicated. Because operator experience is a crucial factor, this technique should be reserved for physicians who are well versed in both sclerotherapy and duplex scanning. When the foregoing principles are implemented by a skilled practitioner, one can expect to obtain consistently satisfactory results with few adverse effects.

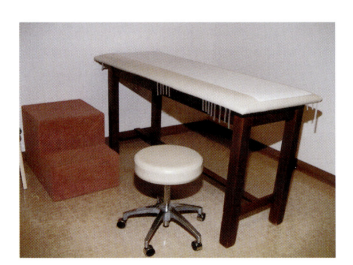

Fig. 14-14. Treatment table (27 × 36 × 72½ in), custom-made cube (20 × 20 in), and adjustable stool. (From Raymond-Martimbeau P: Color atlas of sclerotherapy for varicose and telangiectatic veins, Dallas, 1994, PRM Editions.)

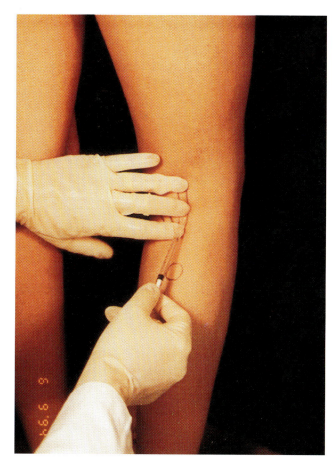

Fig. 14-15.   Injection of the saphenopopliteal junction using the sequestration technique. (From Raymond-Martimbeau P: Color atlas of sclerotherapy for varicose and telangiectatic veins, Dallas, 1994, PRM Editions.)

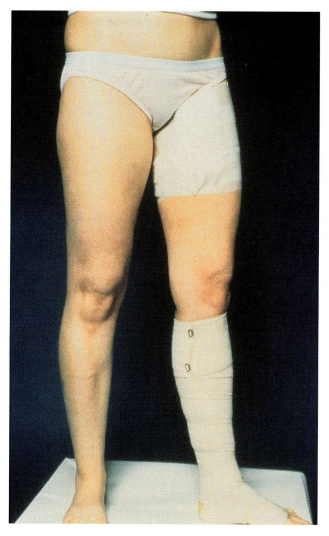

Fig. 14-16.   Postsclerotherapeutic care: selective compressive dressing and elastic bandage. (From Raymond-Martimbeau P: Color atlas of sclerotherapy for varicose and telangiectatic veins, Dallas, 1994, PRM Editions.)

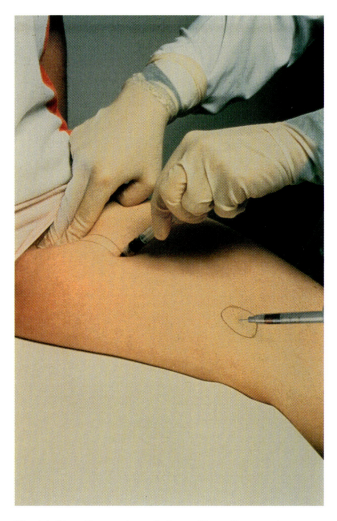

Fig. 14-17. Composite technique. (From Raymond-Martimbeau P: Color atlas of sclerotherapy for varicose and telangiectatic veins, Dallas, 1994, PRM Editions.)

■ References

1. Raymond-Martimbeau P: Color atlas of sclerotherapy for varicose and telangiectatic veins, Dallas, 1994, PRM Editions.

2. Wallois P: Mise à jour de la technique de la suppression des reflux saphéniens par sclérothérapie, Phlébologie 35:337-348, 1982.

3. Wallois P: The conditions necessary to achieve an effective sclerosant treatment, Phlébologie 39:223-226, 1986.

4. Raymond-Martimbeau P: Advanced sclerotherapy treatment of varicose veins with duplex ultrasonographic guidance, Semin Dermatol 12:123-128, 1993.

5. Raymond-Martimbeau P: Anatomy of the venous system of the lower limbs. In Raymond-Martimbeau P, editor: Phlebologia Houston '91, Dallas, 1991, PRM Editions, pp 29-35.

6. Grondin L, Raymond-Martimbeau P: Superficial venous system disorders. In Leclerc JR, editor: Thromboembolic disorders. Philadelphia, 1990, Lea & Febiger, pp 412-429.

7. Raymond-Martimbeau P: Role of sclerotherapy in greater saphenous vein incompetence. In Bergan JJ, Goldman MP, editors: Varicose veins and telangiectasias: diagnosis and treatment, St Louis, 1993, Quality Medical Publishing, pp 226-258.

8. Cloutier G: La sclérose des crosses des saphènes internes et externes: nouvelle approche, Phlébologie 29:227-232, 1976.

9. Cloutier G, Sansoucy H: La sclérose des crosses des saphènes internes et externes avec compression: résultats, Phlébologie 33:731-735, 1980.

10. Cloutier G, Zummo M: La sclérose des crosses avec compression: résultats à long terme, Phlébologie 39:145-148, 1986.

11. Wallois P: Matériel et technique de sclérothérapie, Phlébologie 39:219-222, 1986.

12. Raymond-Martimbeau P: Two different techniques for sclerosing the incompetent saphenofemoral junction: a comparative study, J Dermatol Surg Oncol 16:626-631, 1990.

13. Saglio H: Mon expérience de l'iode, Phlébologie 31:63-66, 1978.

14. Chatard H: A propos de la sclérothérapie des saphènes variqueuses: quelques points de technique, Phlébologie 31:79-83, 1978.

15

MACROSCLEROTHERAPY AND ANGIOSCOPY

Ken P. Biegeleisen

Angioscopic delivery of sclerosant is the most effective sclerosing technique for treating varicose veins. It is the only method that is capable of reliably bringing about sclerosis of greater saphenous varicosities with proximal diameters of 10 mm or larger with a *single injection* of 3% sodium tetradecyl sulfate.[1] Angioscopic injection is probably the safest available technique because that single injection under direct vision virtually obviates the risk of intraarterial accidents.

■ METHOD OF ANGIOSCOPIC INJECTION OF THE GREATER SAPHENOUS VEIN

Angioscopic treatment of varicose veins requires a considerable investment in equipment. Fig. 15-1 shows the equipment we used in our studies. In addition to one or more angioscopes, it is necessary to purchase a light source, an infusion pump, a specialized video-camera, and other ancillary equipment along with these devices. The minimum start-up cost for such a setup was approximately $30,000 at the time of these studies.

Angioscopes come in a variety of sizes and styles. We limited ourselves to angioscopes with external diameters of less than 2 mm. In general, instruments in that size range have a single injection channel and are nonsteerable. Some larger instruments have multiple channels or are steerable, but these features, highly desirable though they are, are only available in instruments that require a surgical incision to insert them into the vein.

The procedure begins by selecting an insertion site. We found it necessary to enter the saphenous trunk itself, which is usually straight. The temptation to enter

large, tortuous surface tributaries must be avoided because they cannot be negotiated with a nonsteerable instrument. We usually attempted to insert the angioscope just above the knee. This is a desirable site because it allows examination of the entire length of the proximal saphenous vein for tributaries, arteriovenous communications, or other vessels into which sclerosant might unintentionally leak and thereby propagate to unintended sites. Most of our procedures were performed with a 1.8 mm angioscope inserted through a 9-French Seldinger catheter. The insertion set is shown in Fig. 15-2, and consists of a guidewire, a dilator, and a sheath.

The leg is thoroughly scrubbed with Betadine, and sterile technique is employed throughout. At first we attempted to perform the insertion with the technique supine. However, even with large-caliber saphenous veins, venospasm often set in, making the procedure impossible to complete. We found that once venospasm set in, it often would not reverse even if we stood the patient up again. Therefore, we ceased attempting angioscopic insertion in any other position than standing.

With the patient standing, a 16-gauge needle without syringe is inserted into the saphenous vein (Fig. 15-3). If a syringe is attached, it should be attached loosely so that it can be removed, and the blood flow through the needle studied. If the blood flow is pulsatile, the needle has entered either the femoral or saphenous artery, and the procedure must be discontinued. Once proper needle placement has been ascertained, the guidewire is passed through the 16-gauge needle into the vein (Fig. 15-4). The needle can then be removed, leaving the guidewire in place (Fig. 15-5).

After the 16-gauge needle is completely separated from the guidewire, we employ its cutting edge as a tiny scalpel to slightly enlarge the insertion point in the skin to approximately 1 mm. The needle is also passed

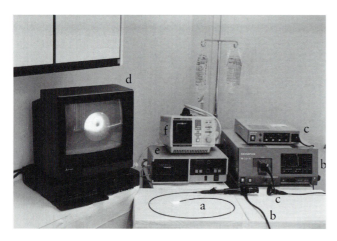

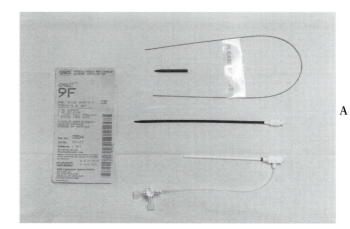

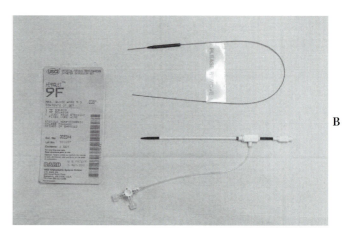

Fig. 15-1. Equipment necessary for venous angioscopy. **A,** Angioscope. This is an Olympus model with a single injection channel. The fluid port is disconnected for the sake of the photograph, but the high-intensity light source (**B**) is connected. The light can be seen emanating from the tip of the angioscope. An angioscopic examination can be monitored visually through the eyepiece. More often, the eyepiece is coupled directly to a tiny video camera, **C.** The camera output goes to a color monitor and video recorder, **D.** Two intravenous infusion setups are desirable. During the steps involved in introducing the angioscope into the vein, it is easiest to work with an ordinary gravity-driven slow infusion, simply to keep the channels of the introducing catheters open. During angioscopic visualization of the vein interior, however, precisely controlled high-speed infusion of fluid is often necessary, which requires that the second infusion be connected to a variable-speed infusion pump, **E.** The model shown (Olympus) is designed especially for angioscopic work and can produce infusions up to 400 cc/minute. Although not absolutely necessary, a good gray-scale ultrasound scanner, **F,** is helpful in guiding the insertion of the first needle into the saphenous trunk. Above the knee, the trunk is rarely visible, and it is highly desirable to avoid inserting the angioscope into the wrong vessel.

Fig. 15-2. **A,** Components of a 9-French Seldinger introduction set. The separate parts (top to bottom) are a guide-wire, a dilator, and a sheath. Each item is required for inserting the next one, and the angioscope itself is inserted through the sheath, as described in the text. **B,** The guide-wire is shown assembled with a small, pointed insertion device, which helps guide it through the needle hub into the shaft. The dilator is inserted into the sheath, and the two together are inserted into the vein, following the path established by the guide-wire, as described in the text.

back into the vein a few times (not over the guidewire but adjacent to it) to enlarge the insertion wound in the vein wall. These steps greatly facilitate the insertion of the dilator and sheath, which would otherwise be difficult to force through the tiny 16-gauge needle-puncture hole. Next, the dilator is put into the 11-French, and the two together are inserted over the guidewire into the vein (Fig. 15-6). A twisting motion is often helpful here. At this point, the patient can be placed on the treatment table in the supine position. The guidewire is withdrawn and a gravity-driven, slow, intravenous infusion can be connected to the dilator to keep the channel patent while the sheath is taped securely to the leg. Once the sheath is taped down, the

dilator can be removed (taking care not to pull out the sheath with it) and the intravenous infusion rerouted to the three-way stopcock of the sheath.

Before inserting the angioscope, it should be laid down on the leg. The length of angioscope necessary to insert to reach the saphenofemoral junction should be estimated in advance. A calibrated instrument is very helpful (Fig. 15-7). The angioscope is next inserted through the sheath into the vein. The pump-driven infusion line is attached to the angioscope infusion port, and the gravity-driven infusion to the triple stopcock can be shut off. The videocamera is attached to the angioscope, and this completes the insertion process.

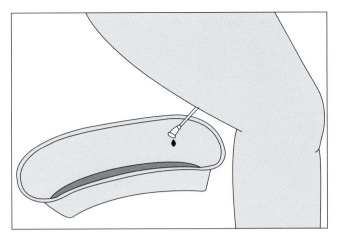

Fig. 15-3. Inserting a 16-gauge needle into the saphenous vein. The flow of blood through the needle is observed. If pulsatile flow is seen, the procedure is discontinued. Note that in this, and in the next three figures, the angle of the needle with respect to the saphenous axis appears nonphysiological, which was done in the interest of graphic clarity.

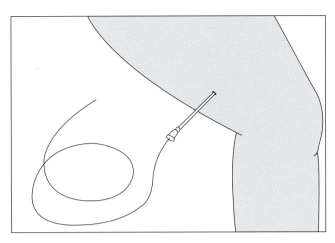

Fig. 15-4. The guide-wire is passed through the needle into the vein.

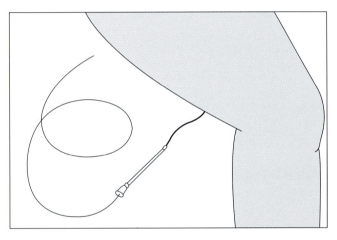

Fig. 15-5. The needle is removed, leaving the guide-wire in place. After the needle is completely disengaged from the guide-wire (not shown), its cutting edge is used to slightly enlarge the insertion wound in the skin. It is then reinserted into the vein, *adjacent* to the guide-wire, to enlarge the puncture wound in the vein wall.

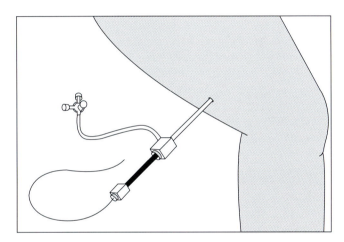

Fig. 15-6. The dilator is inserted into the sheath, and the two together are inserted into the vein, following the guide-wire. A gentle twisting motion is helpful here.

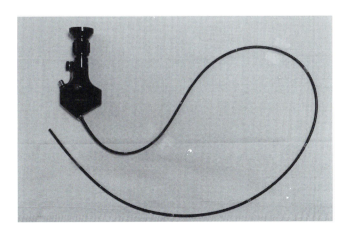

Fig. 15-7. Calibrated fibroscope. Actually this device is a uteroscope (Schott), but it functions very nicely as an angioscope. By laying it on the surface of the patient's leg, the operator can count calibration marks and thereby predetermine how far the device must be inserted to reach the saphenofemoral junction.

■ TECHNIQUE OF ANGIOSCOPIC INJECTION

The most important part of this procedure is identifying the saphenofemoral junction. This is done in three ways:

1. The length of the angioscope necessary to insert should have been estimated beforehand. When this length has been inserted, you should be at or near the junction.

2. The orifices of the proximal saphenous tributaries are readily visible and easily recognized just below the saphenofemoral valve (Fig. 15-8).

3. A bloodless visual field is readily attainable below the saphenofemoral valve, but is impossible to attain above it.

This last point is worth elaborating upon. One unexpected finding of our first angioscopic procedures was the great volume and pressure of reflux through the saphenofemoral junction, making visualizing the junction area difficult. Unless the visual field is cleared of blood by administering intravenous fluid, nothing can be seen. A clear visual field can be obtained *below* the saphenofemoral valve, but not above.

In midthigh, it is often possible to clearly visualize the interior of the saphenous vein with only a minimum infusion of intravenous fluid. As one approaches the saphenofemoral junction, however, the field becomes totally obscured by blood, and no infusion rate (up to 400 cc/minute, the maximum rate possible with the Olympus pump) will clear it. This is true even with the leg elevated to 90 degrees. To see the proximal saphenous vein, it is necessary for an assistant to press forcefully on the saphenofemoral junction from the surface, to physically block reflux. Obviously, this can interfere with full visualization of the most proximal 1 to 2 cm of the saphenous vein in some cases. This is a serious limitation of current angioscopes that will only be overcome by incorporating ultrasound capabilities into these instruments.

The amount of pressure the assistant must apply to prevent reflux through a 10 mm or larger saphenofemoral junction is surprising and is much greater than might be assumed. It turns out that even with the leg at 90 degrees, the proximal saphenous vein is anything but "empty." In fact, it is flooded with rapidly moving blood that, more than anything else, probably accounts for the extreme unreliability of "cross" injection as it is usually performed. The medicine is literally washed away before it can take effect.

In venous angioscopy, the brisk blood flow at the saphenofemoral junction can be employed as an anatomic marker, to ascertain that the tip of the angio-

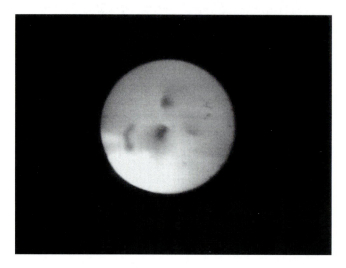

Fig. 15-8. Angioscopic view of the saphenofemoral junction (high-resolution video print). An assistant, pressing from the surface, has caused the lumen of the vein (center of the print) to be pressed nearly flat. Arrayed about the lumen, at the 12, 3, and 9 o'clock positions, the orifices of the proximal saphenous tributaries are clearly seen. A bit of blood floating upward from the 9 o'clock tributary gives it an elongated look. If the angioscope were advanced just beyond the tributary orifices, the saphenous valve cusps would be clearly visible. They are not visible in this view because of the assistant's manual compression of the saphenofemoral junction. If this compression is gradually released, it is usually possible to see the valve cusps briefly, before the visual field becomes totally obscured by retrograde blood flow.

scope is just below the saphenofemoral valve (the preferred site for injection). Above the valve, no amount of intravenous fluid or surface pressure will yield a bloodless field while below the valve, a bloodless field is almost always attainable by a brisk infusion of intravenous fluid combined with firm digital pressure on the saphenofemoral junction from the surface. We generally pass the angioscope up and back across the valve several times until we are absolutely certain that the tip lies just below it.

Once the location of the angioscope tip has been confirmed, the intravenous infusion is disconnected. A syringe containing 3% sodium tetradecyl sulfate is attached to the injection port of the angioscope. A volume of medicine between 2 and 5 cc (depending on the size of the vessel) is injected while the angioscope is being withdrawn, to distribute the medicine along the length of the vein. The volume can be safely injected because there is no possibility whatsoever of being in an artery and not knowing it, and because the assistant's manual pressure from the surface prevents medicine from passing proximally into the femoral vein. Furthermore, the interior of the saphenous vein is clearly observed through the angioscope during its trip up to the junction. if there are any major tributaries through which sclerosant can migrate to unintended sites, these will be known in advance, and the injected volume can be reduced accordingly. There were no cases of this in the patients we treated, however.

The single most important aspect of this injection is *control of reflux through the saphenofemoral junction at the moment of injection.* In all our cases in which reflux *was* successfully controlled by digital pressure by the assistant (indicated by a clear visual field), a single angioscopic injection brought about complete sclerosis of the saphenous vein, at least down to the point of insertion of the angioscope.[1] On the other hand, when the angioscopic injection *failed* to sclerose the vein, retrospective inspection of the operative notes revealed that the assistant had lost control of the junction and that the first injection had been made into a bloody field. This resulted in treatment failure, surely due to dilution and "washing away" of the injected medication.

After the angioscope is withdrawn, there will be a brisk bleeding from the insertion site in most cases. This can be successfully controlled by firm manual pressure for a few minutes. The insertion site is then taped, one or more cottonballs taped over it, and a firm compression dressing applied (tape over a layer of cast padding). Once the proximal saphenous trunk has been sclerosed, any residual varicosities can be injected by ordinary compression sclerotherapy on the return office visit.

RESULTS

We attempted angioscopic sclerotherapy on a total of 18 veins in 16 patients. In four cases, we failed to insert the angioscope. In the other cases, however, the short-term results were excellent.[1] Of the 14 veins into which the angioscope was successfully inserted, 12 were found to be totally sclerotic from the saphenofemoral junction at least down to the angioscope insertion site. This was determined by ultrasound examination employing a color-flow triplex scanner. Both of the two treatment failures were cases where control of reflux through the saphenofemoral junction had been lost at the moment of injection so that the medication was injected into a bloody field. Therefore, in 12 of 12 cases in which the injection was made into a *bloodless* field, there was complete sclerosis of the proximal saphenous vein with a *single injection.* In our experience, such uniformity and reliability in results is not imaginable with conventional blind-surface injections, even if they are done under ultrasound guidance.

Thus, the short-term result of angioscopic sclerotherapy is far superior to any other injection method we have employed. Although the procedure is cumber-

some and time-consuming, the amount of time spent with the patient in the long-run is actually less than the total time spent in repeatedly injecting "blindly" into the saphenofemoral area over a period of three to six office visits (which is what we had previously found to be necessary employing "conventional" injection methods). The long-term result, however, was recanalization. Each of the 12 successfully sclerosed veins recanalized by the end of the first year.

THE PROMISE OF ANGIOSCOPY

Three technical problems must be overcome before angioscopy will replace ordinary injections and surgery:

1. Ultrasound capabilities must be incorporated into existing angioscope designs. There are many sites in the venous system where high flow renders it impossible to obtain a clear visual field. The saphenofemoral injection, when it is grossly varicose, is one such site. These cases should be managed by ultrasound visualization. Pure ultrasound-imaging catheters now exist, but because so much of venous medicine involves low-flow areas as well as high-flow areas, pure ultrasound catheters would be even more inadequate than pure fiberoptic catheters. A catheter with both modalities is needed.

2. Steerability must be developed for instruments of less than 2 to 2 mm in outer diameter. The varicosities system is full of sharp curves and turns even when normal. In varicosities, the tortuosity makes it even worse. Without a steerable instrument, one is limited to procedures involving straight segments of vein. At the time we performed the studies described here, the smallest steerable instrument we found had an outer diameter of 1.8 mm, but it had no injection channel. The addition of an injection channel, using current technology, results in a device so large that surgery is required to insert it. It might logically be argued that once the procedure is started surgically, it might as well be finished surgically, thus obviating the need for angioscopy in the first place.

3. Better medicines or alternative nonpharmacologic therapies must be perfected.

Through the modality of venous angioscopy, it may become possible to perform treatments that are rarely even thought of currently, much less done. As one example, I would cite the possibility of sparing the saphenous trunk by obliteration of the arteriovenous communications.[6]

Starting with our very first angioscopic venous procedure, and regularly ever since, we have directly

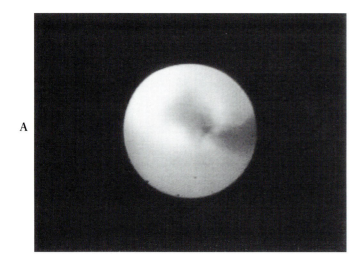

A

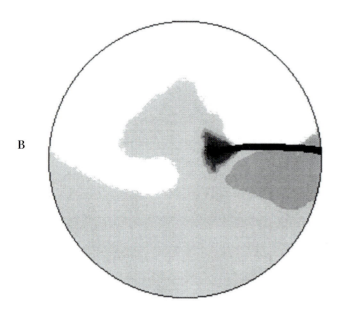

B

observed orifices of small, pulsatile tributary vessels in the trunk of the greater saphenous vein (Fig. 15-9). By virtue of the venous angioscope, it may soon be possible to selectively obliterate these tiny pulsatile vessels by injection, electrocautery, or laser without damage to the saphenous trunk itself. If the arteriovenous theory of the etiology of varicose veins is correct, such a procedure might "cure" the saphenous vein of varicose disease and completely spare the trunk for later use as a conduit in arterial bypass surgery.

Acknowledgements

These studies were made possible by the generous provision of angioscopes and ancillary equipment by Olympus (Japan) and Schott (Germany).

■ REFERENCES

1. Biegeleisen K, Nielsen RD: Failure of angioscopically guided sclerotherapy to permanently obliterate greater saphenous varicosity, Phlebology 9(1):21-24, 1994.

2. Hobbs JT: Surgery and sclerotherapy in the treatment of varicose veins, Arch Surg 109:793-796, 1974.

3. Kunnen M, Comhaire F: Transcatheter embolization of the internal spermatic vein(s) with Bucrylate: further improvements, Ann Radiol 27:303, 1984.

4. Libutti SK, Oz MC, Chuck RS, Treat MR, Nowygrod R: Dye-enhanced tissue welding using fibrinogen and continuous-wave argon lasers, Vasc Surg 24(9):671-676, 1990.

5. Schalin L: Arteriovenous communications to varicose veins in the lower extremities studied by dynamic angiography, Acta Chir Scand 146:397-406, 1980.

6. Schalin L: Arteriovenous communications in varicose veins localized by thermography and identified by operative microscopy, Acta Chir Scand 147:409-420, 1981.

Fig. 15-9. Arteriovenous communication (avc) in the trunk of the greater saphenous vein; angioscopic view. This is a high-resolution print of a freeze frame from a video. In motion, the avc is quite dramatic, demonstrating a prominent visual pulsation with each heartbeat. On a freeze frame like this, however, we were somewhat dismayed to find that it was barely visible. Therefore we produced a graphic recreation, **B**, showing the location of the avc as a bold black line emanating from the 3 o'clock position and extending inward toward the lumen of the vessel. If you look back at **A**, you will now see the avc, although it is very faint. We saw this particular avc on the first venous angioscopy we ever did and have seen them regularly ever since.

16

MACROSCLEROTHERAPY AND DUPLEX TECHNOLOGY

Vin Frederic and Michel Schadeck

Ultrasound-guided sclerotherapy is the logical result of combining macrosclerotherapy and duplex technology and consists of monitoring and guiding the injection of sclerosant in varices by duplex scanning. Ultrasound-guided macrosclerotherapy was first proposed in 1989 for treating superficial venous networks and making the injection safely.[1] This is often difficult because of a small size, an important depth, and a non-palpable vein.[2]

Materials include a good duplex scanner with high-frequency probe, a soft-plastic syringe, a needle of appropriate length (1½ inches), and a small angiocatheter.[3] The echomographic examination can be made in longitudinal or transversal section (Fig. 16-1). The vein has to be completely compressed by the probe to differentiate it from an artery. For arteries, compressing the vessel enhances pulsations. The size of the vein and depth of the posterior wall are measured so the physician can choose a needle of appropriate length. These measurements must be made with the patient in the supine position. Fill the syringe with appropriate sclerosing agent (frequently sodium tetradecyl sulfate). Take the probe in one hand and the syringe in the other. In the transversal section, we place the cross-section area of the vein in the center of the screen and the needle in the middle of the probe (Fig. 16-2). In the longitudinal section, the vein appears clearly on the screen. The needle is placed in the middle of the other side of the probe (Fig. 16-3). When the extremity of the needle is strictly in the lumen of the vein, it appears distinctly on the screen as a white point only if it is in the cross-section of the probe. Blood is aspirated into the syringe (Fig. 16-4).

The injection is made slowly and the reflux is frequently verified. During the injection, we observe on the screen white echoes corresponding to the sclerosing agent and sometimes to small bubbles of air. After the injection, compression can be placed on the leg depending on the level of the injection. In certain cases (such as the lesser saphenous vein), we make an open incision with a microcatheter (Fig. 16-5).[3]

◼ INDICATIONS

Anterior Saphenous Vein

(Fig. 16-6) The anterior saphenous vein is an excellent indication for ultrasound-guided sclerotherapy. Duplex examination shows the anterior saphenous vein in front of the femoral artery. Ultrasound-guided injection reduces the risk of arterial injection. We start the treatment using sodium tetradecyl sulfate (STS) 3%, 1 cc for a diameter less than 5 mm and 2 cc for a diameter greater than 8 mm.

Greater Saphenous Vein

(Fig. 16-7) Frequently, injection of the sapheno-femoral injection is easy. Sometimes with significant reflux, the diameter is too small and the clinical palpation is difficult. In this case, ultrasound-guided sclerotherapy is also an excellent indication. When the diameter of the greater saphenous vein is small and reflux is minimal, we recommend one injection 5 cm distal to the injection (STS 3%, 1 cc for diameter less than 5 mm and 2 cc for diameter greater than 5 mm.[4,5] When the saphenous trunk is large, greater than 5 to 6 mm, we recommend making two injections: the first at the junction as proposed earlier and the second on the middle of the thigh with STS 1% to 1.5%, 1 to 2 cc.

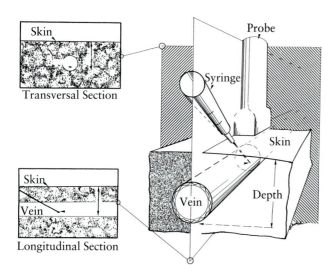

Fig. 16-1. Principle of ultrasound-guided sclerotherapy in longitudinal and transversal sections.

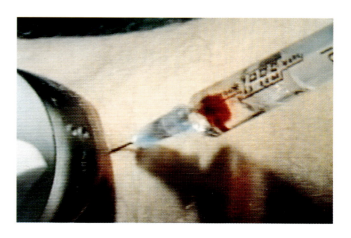

Fig. 16-4. Reflux of blood in the syringe.

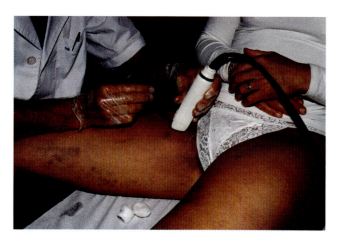

Fig. 16-2. Sclerotherapy of the greater saphenous vein in longitudinal section.

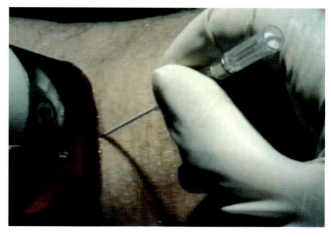

Fig. 16-5. Using a minicatheter in the treatment of a lesser saphenous vein.

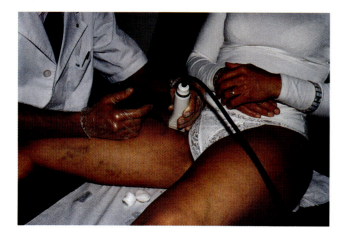

Fig. 16-3. Sclerotherapy of the greater saphenous vein in transversal section.

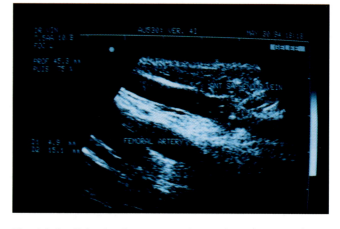

Fig. 16-6. Injection into an anterior saphenous vein in longitudinal section.

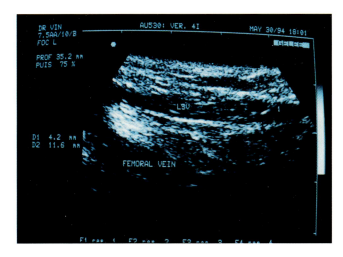

Fig. 16-7. Injection into a greater saphenous vein in longitudinal section. We observed the echoes of the sclerosing agent during this injection.

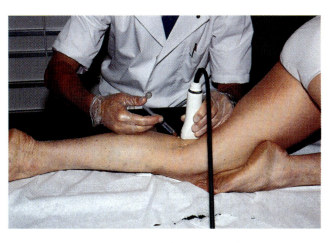

Fig. 16-8. Kneeling position of the patient during injection of the lesser saphenous vein in the transversal section.

Lesser Saphenous Vein

The complexity of the saphenopopliteal junction, the possibility for different connections with gastrocnemius veins, and the proximity of various arteries call for special precautions.[6] All veins less than 9 mm in diameter can be injected. The patient can be placed in two different positions, the prone position or the kneeling position. In the prone position (Fig. 16-8), the lesser saphenous vein is often flattened and difficult to inject. In the kneeling position, the vein is open and access is easier. Avoid placing the needle in the wall because of the risk of extravasation (Fig. 16-9). It is possible to use a minicatheter when the patient is in the prone position and inject safely. However, the catheter has to be sufficiently rigid because the wall is often very resistant and can cause the catheter to deviate. We start treatment with STS 3%, 1 cc in the popliteal fold after verifying neighboring vessels. For large lesser saphenous veins 5 to 9 mm, we can make another injection in the middle of the calf and place appropriate compression.

Perforating Veins

Perforating veins can be treated in isolation when no other sites of venous incompetence exist (Fig. 16-10). The anatomy of perforating veins is variable. There are three principal levels: in the midthigh, medial knee, and medial calf and ankle. The concern when injecting perforating veins is the proximity to the arterial and deep-vein systems. When injecting, it is best to place the needle into the varicose veins in front of the perforator or in the distal extremity of the perforator. We start of treatment with STS, 1.5%, 1 cc at the thigh;

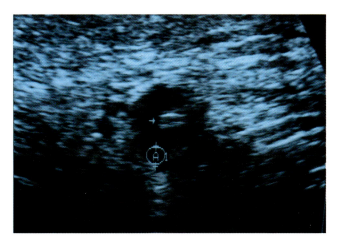

Fig. 16-9. Lesser saphenous vein in transversal section. Just below the vein observe (circle and **A**) the satellite artery of this vein.

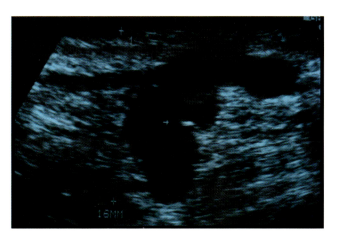

Fig. 16-10. Injection into a large Cockett's perforator. The white point represents the extremity of the needle.

1%, 1 cc at the knee level; and 0.5%, 1 cc at the calf and ankle region.

Postsurgical Recurrences

Post surgical recurrences are often considered by many authors to be the ideal indication for ultrasound-guided sclerotherapy (Fig. 16-11).[8] At the common femoral vein level, we sometimes find a stump with small refluxing branches. In other cases, we can see neogenesis with angioma around the common femoral vein. With the duplex, we can inject sclerosant into the small vessels to stop the reflux. At the popliteal fossa level, we see a similar appearance with incompetence of gastrocnemius perforators. The sclerosing agent is more effective for the new vessels that have thin walls. We recommend STS, 0.5% to 1%, 1 to 2 cc.

Obesity

Obesity is certainly one of the best indications of ultrasound-guided sclerotherapy (Fig. 16-12). The depth of the vein above 20 mm makes palpation impossible. With "echoguidance," sclerotherapy is easier.[9] We have to measure the depth of the posterior wall of the vein and choose a needle of appropriate length.

■ COMPLICATIONS

Minor complications are found in all sclerosing injections.[10] Hematoma, inflammatory reactions, and extravascular injections can be seen on the screen (Fig. 16-13). Sometimes injections in the venous wall with a bubble in the lumen can be seen (Fig. 16-14). Major complications of anaphylactic shock, arterial or arteriolar injections,[11] and open needle insertion into the vein are avoided with "echocontrol" and clinical experience. Deep-venous thrombosis has not occurred in our practice even when we see the sclerosing agent slowly moving toward the deep-venous system.

■ SUMMARY

Ultrasound-guided sclerotherapy has added to the phlebologist's therapeutic arsenal. It consists of monitoring and guiding (by duplex) the injection of sclerosing agents into varicose veins. The aim is to make the injection safely and avoid extravasation and arterial injection. It can also treat superficial venous networks not palpable with clinical examination. With this new method, it is possible to treat the varicose veins reflux points at their origin.

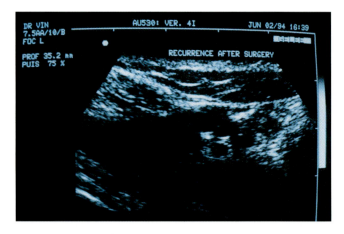

Fig. 16-11. Stump of the greater saphenous vein and the injection inside.

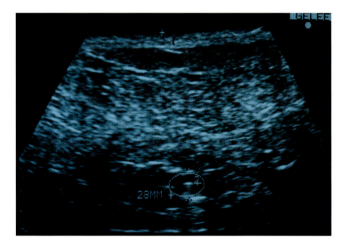

Fig. 16-12. Injection of a "small" greater saphenous vein (3.5 mm size and 28 mm depth) in an obese patient.

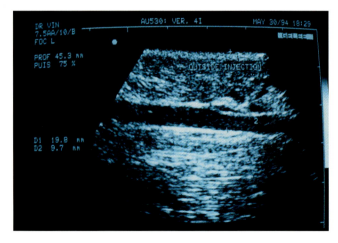

Fig. 16-13. Injection outside the lumen.

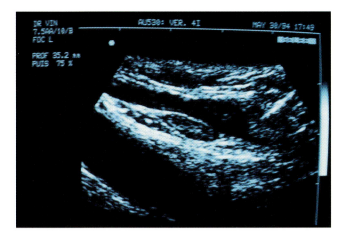

Fig. 16-14.   Injection in the wall gives a bubble in the lumen.

■ REFERENCES

1. Knight RM, Vin F, Zygmunt JA: Ultrasonic guidance of injection into the superficial venous system. In Davy A, Stemmer R, editors: Phlebologie '89, Paris, 1989, John Libbey Eurotext, Ltd, pp 339-41.

2. Knight RM: Treatment of superficial venous disease with accurate sclerotherapy, Proc Can Soc Phlebol, Whistler, 1991.

3. Grondin L: Personal communication, 1993.

4. Forestal M, Foley D, Birnholz J: Sclerotherapy of truncal greater and/or lesser saphenous veins with duplex ultrasound guidance. Proc Can Soc Phlebol, Whistler, 1991.

5. Schadeck M. Echosclerose de la grande saphene: Methodologie et resultats, Phlebologie 46:673-82, 1993.

6. Vin F: Echosclerotherapie de la veine saphene externe, Phlebologie 44:79-84, 1991.

7. Thibault PK, Lewis WA: Recurrent varicose veins. Part 2: Injection of incompetent perforating veins ultrasound guidance, J Dermatol Surg Oncol 18:895-900, 1992.

8. Vin F: Echosclerotherapy of recurrent varicose veins after surgery. In Raymond-Martimbeau P, Prescott R, Zummo M, editors: Phlebologie '92, Paris, John Libbey Eurotext, pp 827.

9. Schadeck M: Duplex and Phlebology. Napoli (ed). Liviana Medicina, 1994 (in press).

10. Grondin L, Soriano J: Echosclerotherapy: a Canadian study. In Raymond-Martimbeau P, Prescott R, Zummo M, editors: Phlebologie '92, Paris, John Libbey Eurotext, pp 828-31.

11. Biegeleisen K, Neilsen RD, O'Shaughnessy A: Inadvertent intra-arterial injection complicating ordinary and ultrasound-guided sclerotherapy, J Dermatol Surg Oncol 19:953-58, 1993.

Part IV

Surgical Alternatives to Sclerotherapy

17

AMBULATORY SURGERY OF VARICOSE VEINS

John J. Bergan

Knowledge based upon prospective studies has clarified indications for methods of venous ablation.[1,2] Surgery is chosen rather than sclerotherapy chiefly because of (1) detection of axial reflux in saphenous veins, (2) large size of varicosities, (3) varicosities in medial and/or anterior thigh, and (4) symptomatic aching pain, heaviness, and other discomforts occurring during prolonged standing or prolonged sitting. Other indications include recurrent superficial thrombophlebitis, external bleeding, or eczematoid dermatitis with or without ulceration.[3] Superficial venous ablation can be performed even after deep-venous thrombosis, but utmost caution should be observed to rule out deep-venous occlusion.[4]

Sclerotherapy, as described elsewhere in this volume, is chosen if the main problem is (1) telangiectasias, (2) reticular varicosities, (3) postoperative persistence or recurrence of varicosities, (4) advanced age of patient, or (5) combinations of these.[5]

When surgery is chosen, three goals to be kept in mind in planning treatment are (1) permanent removal of the source of venous hypertension and the varicosities in as (2) cosmetic fashion as possible with a (3) minimum number of complications.[6] The sources of venous hypertension are gravitational (hydrostatic) or compartmental pressure developed during muscular contraction (hydrodynamic). Therefore, correcting gravitational reflux by axial vein removal and detaching hydrodynamic forces by superficial varicosity excision or perforating vein interruption has been found to accomplish the first objective.[7] Experience in treating recurrent varicose veins has revealed that an inadequate procedure at the saphenofemoral junction is a principal finding.[8] This is reemphasized by Darke in Chapter 19. An equally important cause of recurrent varicosities is failure of the primary surgery to remove completely the offending varicosities.

SURGICAL PLAN

The planned operation for a given patient must be completely individualized. Doppler and duplex studies have shown that in 70% of limbs selected for surgery, typical saphenofemoral reflux will be present. In these, the saphenous vein at the femoral junction must be operated upon (Fig. 17-1). However, atypical varicosities without saphenofemoral junction reflux do occur in some 20% of limbs. Others have atypical reflux points causing their varicosities.[9] Clearly, no standard operation fits every patient perfectly.

Techniques of saphenous surgery are well described in standard surgical texts.[10,11] Their outpatient variations are now done routinely.[12,13] This means that older methods requiring inpatient care, general anesthetic, long operating times, radical dissection and ligation of varicose veins, and stripping of saphenous veins to the ankle can be largely abandoned.[14] The operation of removing the saphenous vein (Fig. 17-2) is now done by groin-to-knee downward stripping of the varicose vein.[13,15] Careful attention to total removal of tributaries to the saphenous vein may decrease the incidence of recurrent varicosities (Fig. 17-3). Techniques to decrease hematoma after downward stripping include irrigation or adrenaline and gauze packing of the saphenectomy tunnel.[13,16] Some advocate using tourniquets during saphenous stripping.[17,18] This is shown in Fig. 17-4. Removal of the lesser saphenous vein or proximal refluxing segments of it is illustrated in Fig. 17-5.

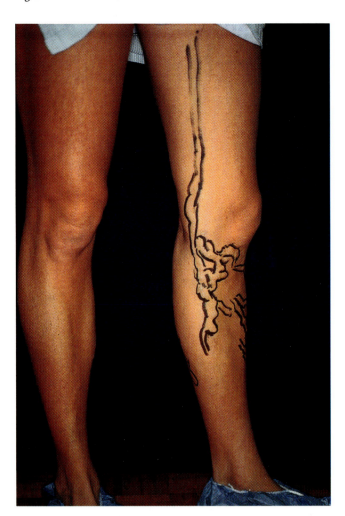

Fig. 17-1.   Carefully marking the varicosities and noting the extent of saphenous vein reflux are an integral part of the ambulatory surgical procedure. In this instance, the saphenous reflux has been detected by Doppler examination, confirmed by duplex, and marked with an indelible felt-tipped pen. Indication of the size and configuration of the varicosities aids in surgically placing the incisions in skin lines to minimize scarring.

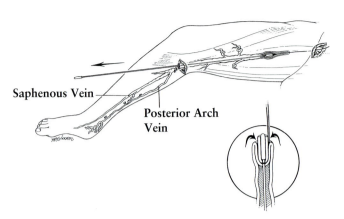

Fig. 17-2.   Principles of inversion stripping of the saphenous vein from above downward are illustrated here. The upper groin incision is made above the inguinal skin crease as indicated by the artist. A heavy ligature is used to fix the upper end of the saphenous vein to the intraluminal stripper, which is removed through a wound exiting in a transverse skin line in the medial aspect of the popliteal fossa. In practice, the ligature is used to draw into the saphenous tunnel a 10 cm gauze strip that has been soaked in adrenaline 1:1,000, one ampule in 250 cc of normal saline. Should the saphenous vein be torn during downward stripping, the gauze pack will pick up the torn segment and deliver it into the distal incision. Important mid- and distal-thigh perforating veins are illustrated by the artist. These maintain patency of the saphenous vein if proximal ligation is performed without stripping. The distal incision can be used to remove anterior tributary varicosities or the upper portion of the posterior arch vein as well as the important anteromedial calf perforating vein of Boyd. Note the location of Cockett perforating veins and their relationship to the posterior arch vein.

■ AMBULATORY PHLEBECTOMY

Various techniques of ambulatory phlebectomy with or without removing the saphenous vein lend themselves to outpatient surgical care. If the phlebectomy is to be combined with saphenous stripping, a word of caution is in order. Greater saphenous stripping often produces proximal venous spasm and distal venous hypertension. Therefore, the endoluminal stripper can be placed early in the operation, but the actual stripping should occur after distal miniphlebectomies are completed. This decreases blood loss markedly.

Miniphlebectomies (Fig. 17-6) can be done with very small incisions (2 to 3 mm), and the varicose vein grasped with one of a variety of small hooks to allow extraction (Fig. 17-7). Clusters of varicosities can be removed, including their perforating connections, without ligation. Reticular varices, reticular veins feeding large telangiectasias, and varicosities draining leg ulcers can be removed using local anesthetic. Unsightly veins in various locations not in the lower extremities can also be removed by miniphlebectomy.[19]

Techniques of hooking varicose veins advocated by Muller, Ramelet, Varady, and others have come into surgical use.[20] Even main saphenous trunks are now subjected to ambulatory phlebectomy, especially by surgeons familiar with the surgical anatomy.[21] However, much care should be exerted in phlebectomy

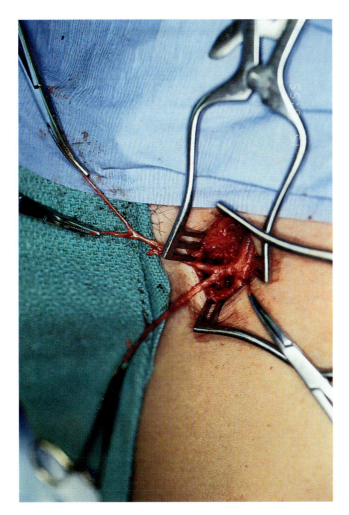

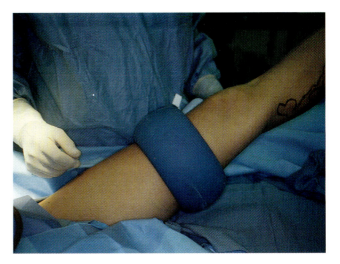

Fig. 17-4. Using the tourniquet considerably decreases blood loss during distal phlebectomy. The Lofqvist tourniquet is illustrated here, but is not available in the United States. The principle of emptying the distal venous tree of enclosed blood and inflating the tourniquet to greater than systolic pressure is a good one and can be accomplished in America by orthopedic tourniquets. The intraluminal stripper can be passed through the saphenous vein under the tourniquet while it is inflated, and sometimes stripping from above downward can be accomplished without deflating the tourniquet. Using the tourniquet eliminates the need for gauze packing of the saphenectomy tunnel.

Fig. 17-3. Tributaries to the saphenous vein are drawn into the surgical incision using traction. The objective is to eliminate from the proximal superficial venous arborization of the primary and even secondary tributaries to the named tributary veins. This will decrease the possibility of residual veins interanastomosing into a network that transmits gravitational reflux distally. The ultimate objective of this maneuver is to decrease late postoperative varicose recurrences.

of the lesser saphenous system because of the intimate relationship of the lesser saphenous vein to the sural nerve.[22]

■ OUTPATIENT SAPHENOUS LIGATION

Economic considerations have forced surgeons to rethink the operation of saphenous ligation. This operation lends itself to outpatient surgery under local anesthetic as illustrated in this volume by Kistner (Chapter 18). It can be performed more easily than saphenous vein stripping. However, experience with outpatient saphenous vein stripping proves that it is easily done without hospitalization and is regularly performed in an outpatient setting.[13]

The fundamental question is what are the results of saphenous-vein ligation alone or in combination with control of varicose clusters. There is now sufficient experience to give a definitive answer. McMullin used noninvasive duplex scanning before and after high ligation of the saphenous vein without stripping in 54 limbs.[23] After operation, duplex scanning revealed that of the 52 limbs in which the saphenofemoral junction had been ligated, there was persistent reflux down the long saphenous vein in 24 cases. His conclusion was that "this operation fails to control functionally significant reflux within the long saphenous vein in a high proportion of cases." Munn showed that significant varicose recurrence is reduced if the saphenous vein is stripped.[24] After proximal ligation without stripping of the saphenous vein, varicography has shown persistent midthigh perforator incompetence in 34%, a patent

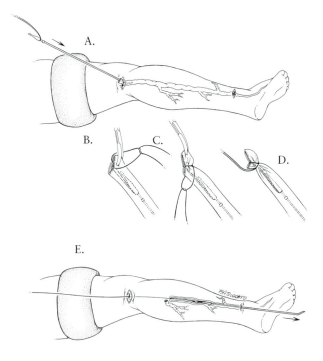

Fig. 17-5. Principles of removing the lesser saphenous vein are illustrated in this figure. Although the Lofqvist tourniquet is illustrated, an orthopedic tourniquet can substitute nicely. The Oesch instrument considerably facilitates proximal-to-distal lesser saphenous removal and is illustrated. The procedure is preceded by careful identification of the termination of the lesser saphenous vein by duplex techniques. This, or intraoperative varicography, is essential to proper placement of the incision because terminating the lesser saphenous vein is exceedingly variable. The steps illustrated in B, C, and D will allow inversion stripping of the lesser saphenous vein whether the Oesch or more readily available instruments are used. As the lesser saphenous vein demonstrates reflux in segments rather than the entire vein, it is most often necessary only to remove the proximal one-third or two-thirds of this vessel, thus avoiding injury to a sural nerve at the ankle. The gauze packing technique referred to earlier can be used in the lesser saphenous system, whether or not the proximal tourniquet is in use.

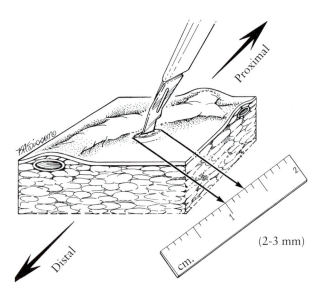

Fig. 17-6. The miniphlebectomy incision is made 2 to 3 mm in length adjacent to, or over, the varicose cluster to be excised. It is placed in skin lines or arbitrarily vertical to avoid lymphatic disruption. Experience teaches that vertical incisions heal with less obvious scars than transverse incisions.

portion of saphenous vein in 54%, and residual or recurrent femoral-saphenous communication in 80%.[25]

In an extensive essay, Neglen compared the operations of ligation alone and ligation and sclerotherapy with stripping of the saphenous vein.[26] High ligation alone was found to be ineffective in controlling varicose recurrence. Similarly, high ligation combined with sclerotherapy or with radical varix removal was inferior to high ligation and stripping of the saphenous vein. Clearly, radical surgery produces the best results in patients with greater saphenous reflux.

Several explanations for this can be found. The first is that duplex ultrasound has shown 70% of limbs studied three years after high ligation have essentially complete preservation of the greater saphenous vein.[27] What happens after high ligation is merely thrombosis to the next tributary vein. If this is the medial posterior tributary, the length of the thrombosed segment will be quite short indeed.

A further argument for segmental saphenous stripping is found in the work of Sutton, who performed retrograde saphenography during saphenous vein surgery.[28] He found varicose changes in 52 of 80 long saphenous veins. The mean length of a normal vein was only 16 cm. More recently, endoscopic evaluation of saphenous veins at the time of saphenous vein surgery has shown the greater saphenous vein in patients with varicosities to be essentially valveless from the groin to just below the knee in 60% of cases.[29] When valves are seen, the intercornual or commissural space allows reflux at the border of valves. This, not the free-valve edge, is found to be the commonest cause of reflux.[30]

Finally, the most recent study of this subject compared saphenofemoral ligation and avulsion of varices with saphenous vein stripping to below the knee and avulsion of varices.[31] When ligation was practiced, 45% of the long saphenous veins in the calf had resid-

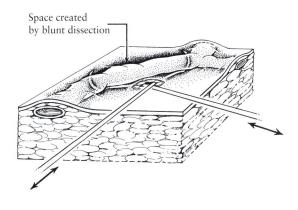

Fig. 17-7. Any one of a variety of hooks can be introduced through the small incision to grasp the underlying varicosity. However, it is important to create space over the vein to be removed using blunt dissection with a small surgical clamp or dissection spatula.

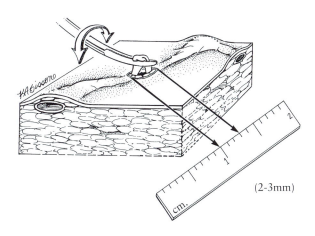

Fig. 17-9. A length of varicosity can be brought through the incision using a rolling or twisting motion and exerting counter-traction on the skin.

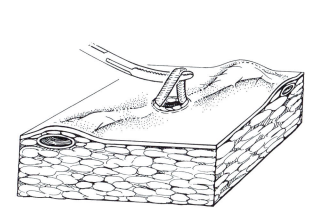

Fig. 17-8. Using the hook allows the varicosity to be brought through the surface of the skin where it can be grasped with a hemostatic clamp.

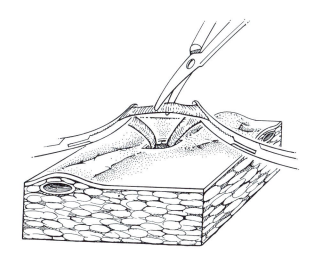

Fig. 17-10. When sufficient length of the varicosity has been brought to the surface, it can be transected and extracted using traction and counter-traction and even identifying primary and secondary tributaries to the cluster.

ual reflux. In contrast, in the group in which the long saphenous vein was stripped, only 18% of the long saphenous veins had reflux which, of course, was limited to the calf. Neither procedure increased the incidence of wound hematoma, wound infection, or paresthesias along the distribution of the saphenous nerve. Adding the stripping of the long saphenous vein in the thigh to multiple avulsions of varicosities resulted in

improving the patient's subjective assessment of the operation. The authors concluded that stripping the long saphenous vein to the upper calf combined with multiple avulsion of varices results in fewer veins with residual reflux and a better functional outcome. Eliminating the option of saphenous ligation with or without distal sclerotherapy or radical varix avulsion simplifies the surgical choice.

■ References

1. Hobbs JT: Surgery and sclerotherapy in the treatment of varicose veins, Arch Surg 109:793-96, 1974.

2. Jakobsen BM: Value of different forms of treatment for varicose veins, Br J Surg 66:182-84, 1979.

3. Tibbs DJ: Varicose veins and related disorders, Oxford, 1992, Butterworth/Heinemann, p 377.

4. Ruckley CV: Surgery for varicose veins, London, 1983, Wolf Medical Publications, Ltd., p 6.

5. Browse NL, Burnand KG, Lea Thomas M: Diseases of the veins, London, 1988, Edward Arnold, p 240.

6. Bergan JJ: Surgical procedures for varicose veins: axial stripping and stab avulsion. In Bergan JJ, Kistner RL, editors: Atlas of venous surgery, Philadelphia, 1992, WB Saunders Co., p 61.

7. Neglen P: Treatment of varicosities of saphenous origin. In Bergan JJ, Goldman MP, editors: Varicose veins and telangiectasias: diagnosis & treatment, St Louis, 1993, Quality Medical Publishers, p 162.

8. Ruckley CV: Surgical management of venous disease, London, 1988, Wolfe Medical Publications, p 56.

9. Goren G, Yellin AE: Primary varicose veins: topographic and hemodynamic correlations, J Cardiovasc Surg 31:672-77, 1990.

10. Lumley JSP: Color atlas of vascular surgery, Baltimore, 1986, Williams & Wilkins.

11. Greenhalgh RM: Vascular surgical techniques, Philadelphia, 1989, WB Saunders Co.

12. Bishop CCR, Jarrett PEM: Outpatient varicose vein surgery under local anaesthesia, Br J Surg 73:821-22, 1986.

13. Bergan JJ: Surgical procedures for varicose veins: axial stripping and stab avulsion. In Bergan JJ, Kistner RL, editors: Atlas of venous surgery, Philadelphia, 1992, WB Saunders Co., p 61-77.

14. Samuels PB: Technique of varicose vein surgery, Am J Surg 142:239-44, 1981.

15. Conrad P: Groin-to-knee downward stripping of the long saphenous vein, Phlebol 7:20-22, 1992.

16. Furuya T, Tada Y, Sato O: A new technique for reducing subcutaneous hemorrhage after stripping of the great saphenous vein, Letter to the Editor, J Vasc Surg 3:493-4, 1992.

17. Corbett R, Jayakumar JN: Clean up varicose vein surgery—use a tourniquet, Ann Royal Col Surg Eng 71:57-8, 1989.

18. Thompson JF, Royle GT, Farrands PA, Najmaldin A, Clifford PC, Webster, JHH: Varicose vein surgery using a pneumatic tourniquet: reduced blood loss and improved cosmesis, Ann Royal Col Surg Eng 72:119-22, 1990.

19. Ramelet AA: La phlebectomie ambulatoire selon muller: technique, avantages, desavantages, J des Maladies Vasculaires 16:119-22, 1991.

20. Chester JF, Taylor RS: Hookers and French strippers: a technique for varicose vein surgery, Br J Surg 77:560-1, 1991.

21. Goren G, Yellin AE: Ambulatory stab evulsion phlebectomy for truncal varicose veins, Am J Surg 162:166-74, 1991.

22. Muller R: Traitement de la saphene externe variqueuse par la phlebectomie ambulatoire, Phlebologie 44:687-92, 1991.

23. McMullin GM, Coleridge-Smith PD, Scurr JH: Objective assessment of ligation without stripping the long saphenous vein, Br J Surg 78:1139-42, 1991.

24. Munn SR, Morton JB, Macbeth WA, McLeish AR: To strip or not to strip the long saphenous vein? a varicose vein trial. Br J Surg 68:426-8, 1981.

25. Corbett CR, Runcie JJ, Lea Thomas M, Jamieson CW: Reasons to strip the long saphenous vein, Phlebologie 41:766-9, 1988.

26. Neglen P: Treatment of varicosities of saphenous origin: comparison of ligation, sclerotherapy, and selected stripping. In Bergan JJ, Goldman MP, editors: Varicose veins & telangiectasias: diagnosis & management, St Louis, 1993, Quality Medical Publishing, Inc.

27. Rutherford RB, Sawyer JD, Jones DN: The fate of residual saphenous vein after partial removal or ligation. J Vasc Surg 12:422-28, 1990.

28. Sutton R, Darke SG: Stripping the long saphenous vein: peroperative (sic) retrograde saphenography in patients with and without venous ulceration, Br J Surg 73:305-7, 1986.

29. Gradman WS: Venoscopy in varicose vein surgery: initial experience. Personal communication.

30. Van Cleef JF, Hugentobler JP, Desvaux P, Griton Ph, Cloarec M. Etude endoscopique des reflux valvulaires sapheniens: J des Maladies Vasculaires 17:113-6, 1992.

31. Sarin S, Scurr JH, Coleridge Smith PD: Assessment of stripping the long saphenous vein in the treatment of primary varicose veins. Br J Surg 79:889-93, 1992.

18

Saphenofemoral Venous Ligation Combined with Sclerotherapy in Treatment of Varicose Veins

Robert L. Kistner and Bo Eklof

Varicose veins can be treated in a number of ways including ligation and stripping, ligation and sclerotherapy, and sclerotherapy alone. Each method has advantages and disadvantages, and it is up to the surgeon to tailor the treatment to the individual case (see Box 18-1).[1] In evolving our approach to this problem, we experienced more than 400 cases treated by saphenofemoral venous ligation and simultaneous sclerotherapy of the varices during a five-year period in the late 1980s. This is the basis upon which we present this technique as an alternative method that may be chosen for selected cases, knowing its advantages and accepting the disadvantages it offers when compared with other methods of treating varicose veins and incompetent greater saphenous veins (GSV).

The reasons to consider high ligation with sclerotherapy are that it is a technically simple surgical means to eliminate the source of direct reflux at the saphenofemoral junction and is a nonsurgical way to eradicate the varices.[2] It can be readily done in an outpatient office surgical setting in a single visit, and the patient can literally walk away from the operating table with a minimum of discomfort. It does not require premedication, and after the procedure a simple analgesic controls the expected discomfort. The patient usually does not return to work the day of surgery, but is able to do self-care entirely, and highly motivated patients are back at work (nonlabor) within three days (Table 18-1).

Using proximal ligation rather than stripping to control axial reflux in the GSV leaves the GSV in place. That the GSV remains as a patent conduit in the majority of instances following ligation with sclerotherapy has been shown by duplex scan studies.[3-5] Of the several theoretical advantages to preserving the GSV over removing the vein, the major one is its preservation as

a future bypass conduit. Although its usefulness for this has not been proved by any published large experience, it would depend upon the condition of the GSV itself because the grossly aneurysmal varicose saphenous vein would not be acceptable either in the heart or in the periphery as a bypass conduit. In most cases the GSV itself is not universally affected by dilation and degeneration, and much if not all of it could be used for bypass.

The major disadvantage to ligation and sclerotherapy is that there is a greater recurrence rate with this technique than occurs after ligation and stripping of the GSV.[6,7]

The treatment that is most reliable for preventing recurrence of varicose veins is the proximal ligation of the GSV at the saphenofemoral junction combined with stripping the saphenous vein at least to the upper-calf level and locally removing the varicosities by separate incisions. This is popularly done now by the technique of outpatient ligation and stripping of the GSV in the thigh and across the knee combined with stab avulsion phlebectomy of the varices themselves.[8] With the physical removal of the varices and stripping of the GSV, recurrences are usually smaller than after other treatments, and they tend to appear 5 to 10 years after the surgery rather than the more frequent 3 to 5 year recurrences seen after ligation with sclerotherapy.

LIGATION AND SCLEROTHERAPY

Our technique for ligation and sclerotherapy is not entirely the same as might be done elsewhere, but it has produced satisfactory results. Both procedures of ligation and sclerotherapy are carried out in a single sitting. There is no formal preparation in the sense of

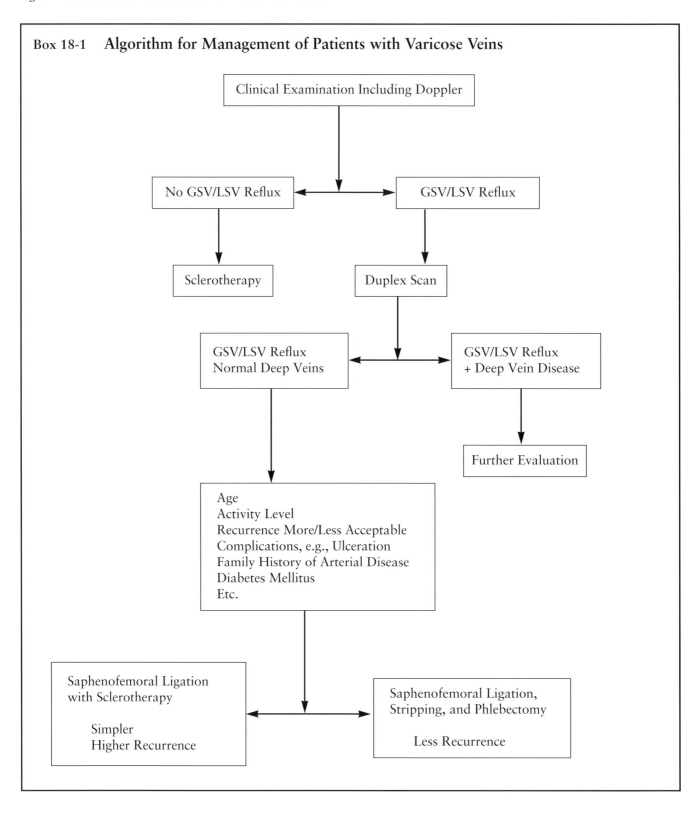

Box 18-1   Algorithm for Management of Patients with Varicose Veins

pretreatment medications or fasting. If a well-equipped outpatient operating room is available where sterile technique can be achieved, going to the hospital operating room is not necessary.

The sclerotherapy is done prior to the ligation because the varices are more prominent in the presence of a refluxing GSV. If the ligation is done first, the varices become less prominent and can be missed at the time of later sclerotherapy, thereby requiring a second injection treatment later when the varices reappear.

Our routine is to have the individual stand next to the operating table to mark the varices. We perform

Table 18-1   High Ligation with Sclerotherapy

Advantages:	Technically simple and safe
	Outpatient
	Single visit
	No premedication
	Patient walks out of OR
	Minimal postoperative pain
	Back to work in 3 days
	Preserves GSV for potential use as arterial bypass
	Reasonable cost
Disadvantages:	Recurrence rate greater than stripping
	Cost and complexity greater than sclerotherapy alone

the sclerotherapy with the patient standing, then have the patient lie down on the operating table while we place a pressure dressing over the sclerosed veins. In that same position, the femoral area is prepped and draped, and formal ligation of the saphenous vein at the saphenofemoral junction is performed under local anesthetic. The dressing is completed after the surgical ligation, the patient rests for a few minutes, then ambulates in the office. The patient is sent home with instructions to keep the pressure dressing on and to ambulate freely.

The patient returns 24 or 48 hours after the procedure to have the leg inspected and to have any questions answered about the routine of wearing firm compression. At this visit the leg is checked to be sure all the varices were treated. Any that have persisted are injected, and the leg is rewrapped to be sure the pressure dressing is properly applied. If there are any prominent hematomas at injection sites, they can be aspirated, but this is rarely needed if a good pressure dressing was applied during the procedure. We have found the pressure dressing to be an integral part of the procedure and consider its use a necessity to achieve optimal results of minimal bruising, good collapse of the treated veins, and minimal hemosiderin staining.

◼ Method of Sclerotherapy

There are many variations of technique for sclerotherapy, and our method varies from the usual in that the actual sclerotherapy is done with the patient standing. Our choice for the sclerosant solution has been sodium tetradecyl sulfate (STS) in various dilutions that are dictated by the varix being treated. The 1% solution is used for all significant-size varices (larger than 2 mm) and has been adequate even for

large varices in our experience, so we have not used the 3% solution. For small superficial varices and reticular veins, we use 0.5% STS. A 0.25% solution is used for telangiectases. The dilutions are made at the bedside by diluting the 1% solution with sterile normal saline. The 0.25% solution has been safe in the dermal tissues when the injection escapes outside the lumen of the vein; in this dilution we have not found skin sloughs to occur. Some sclerotherapists advocate dilution to 0.1% for the very superficial and delicate telangiectases.[9] Controlled experiments are now being reported that demonstrate less staining with polidocanol than with STS,[10] and this may become the standard of therapy in the future.

Sclerotherapy for this procedure is generally limited to large-size veins for which we employ the STS 1% solution. For an average-size adult we use as much as 15 ml of solution at one sitting without experiencing side effects. Each injection consists of 1 ml of solution in a given site.

With the patient standing, the injections are performed by palpating the previously marked vein, inserting the #26 needle, aspirating blood to be certain the needle is in the lumen, and injecting 1 ml into the vein (Fig. 18-1). If the injectate begins to extravasate, the injection is stopped, and the needle replaced into the lumen. Pressure is manually applied by an assistant with a folded 2 × 2 pledget immediately over the injection site for 30 or more seconds to fix the injectate to the endothelium. Multiple injections are made (Fig. 18-2) throughout the extremity to treat all of the varices present in one session whenever possible.

The patient is then asked to lie supine on the operating table, and a carefully applied pressure dressing is performed using foam padding (¼ inch) cut to the course of the individual varices, held in place with gently placed small tape strips, and wrapped with at least two layers of elastic bandage from the foot to the highest level of sclerotherapy (Fig. 18-3). This bandage remains in place until the first postoperative visit on day 1, 2, or 3, when it is replaced by a similar bandage that is left in place for one week.

In the second week the bandage can be replaced by a well-fitted surgical knee-length compression stocking of 30 to 40 mmHg compression. After 2 to 3 weeks pressure is no longer required unless the patient has complicated venous insufficiency or is healing an ulcer.

This technique of sclerotherapy is quick to perform, effective in providing reliable obliteration of varices, and cosmetically acceptable. Using the standing position for injection permits rapid placement of needles into the lumen, certain placement of the solution inside the lumen because blood can be aspirated whenever there is doubt that the solution is going intraluminal, and reliable retention of the solution at the site because the patient is standing and venous flow is static.

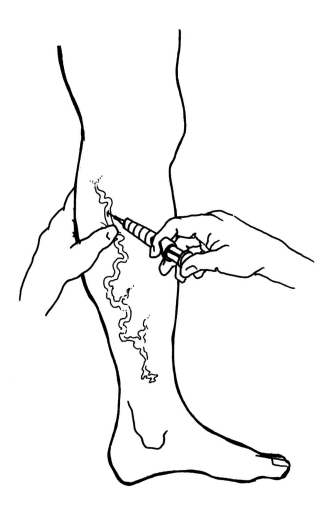

Fig. 18-1. Sclerotherapy. Direct venipuncture with the patient erect.

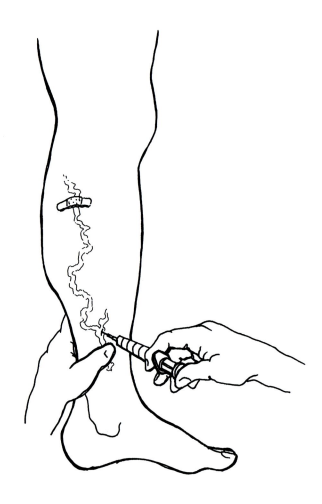

Fig. 18-2. Sclerotherapy. Multiple injections placed sequentially.

Pressure over the injection site with a folded 2 × 2 pledget for 30 seconds allows interaction of the solution with the intima, and we find this is adequate time to initiate the process of intimal destruction. It has been shown that endothelial damage begins within one second of exposure to detergent solutions such as STS.[9]

We have not found it necessary to place the needle when the patient is standing and then have the patient lie down before injection to obtain an effective sclerosing effect. It is faster to do the injections with the patient standing, and it is more certain to place all of the solution inside the vein when one can aspirate during injection to check the position of the needle. This technique allows treatment of many different sites at one sclerotherapy session. It is important to be mindful that some patients will develop a vasovagal reaction and become faint in the vertical position; if this occurs the patient must lie down before syncope occurs. After a short rest period the process can be resumed; faintness seldom happens a second time.

The pressure dressing is an integral part of the treatment and an absolute necessity for achieving good results. If the dressing does not collapse the vein and remain in place, there will be a good chance that either an intraluminal hematoma will form or the varix will not be obliterated. This is the purpose of the early visit on day 1 or 2 after the procedure when the pressure dressing can be checked and corrected if need be. At this time further injections can be done to treat the occasional missed varix, and, if there are any significant hematomas, they can be aspirated.

METHOD OF SAPHENOFEMORAL LIGATION

With the patient in the supine position and the extremity wrapped in a pressure dressing over the sites of

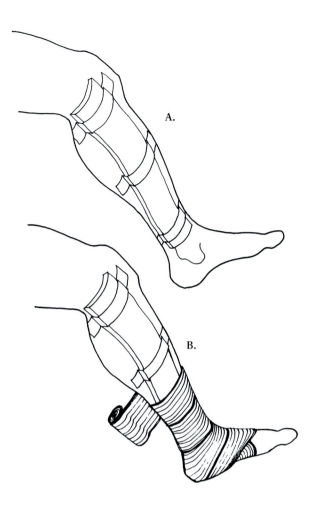

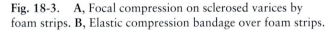

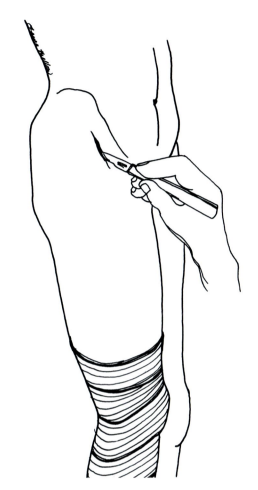

Fig. 18-3.   A, Focal compression on sclerosed varices by foam strips. B, Elastic compression bandage over foam strips.

Fig. 18-4.   Skin-line incision for saphenofemoral vein ligation under local anesthesia.

sclerotherapy, the femoral area is prepped and draped under sterile technique. We have found the procedure to be sufficiently gentle that sedation is seldom necessary, and this allows the alert patient to cooperate with all of the steps in the procedure.

The ligation is performed through a skin-line incision in the inguinal skin crease with the lateral aspect of the incision at the site of the femoral pulse (Fig. 18-4). The GSV is identified in the subcutaneous tissue, elevated from its bed, and transected when its identification is certain. The distal end is inspected for large tributaries, and if any are found they are separately ligated and divided. The distal end of the GSV is ligated and suture-ligated to ensure that the tie will not come off during the healing process when the patient is an outpatient. We inject 4 cc of 1% STS in the distal divided stump of the GSV to discourage late neovascularization.

The proximal divided stump of the GSV is used as a sort of handle with a clamp in place on the stump to facilitate identification of all vein branches down to the saphenofemoral junction. Each branch is dissected locally and ligated and transected as far from the main trunk as can be readily reached to discourage late neovascularization (Fig. 18-5).

The common femoral vein (CFV) is carefully and thoroughly exposed to be certain of its correct identification and to ligate any branches of the CFV in this vicinity. The saphenous vein is transected and ligated flush with the CFV (Fig. 18-6). This is important to minimize recurrences in the late postoperative follow-up.

Closure of the wound is done in layers after hemostasis is complete (Fig. 18-7). If hematomas are avoided, there are seldom any complications of this dissection, and usually there is no pain. In most cases the scar becomes invisible in late follow-up.

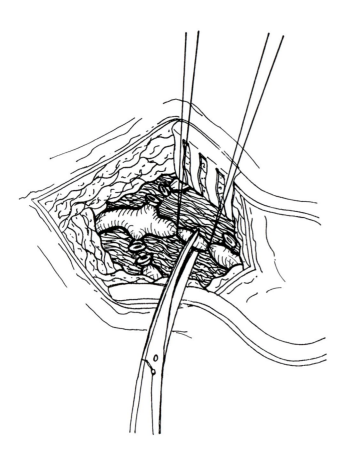

Fig. 18-5. Division of GSV in the line of the incision and ligation of distal end of GSV.

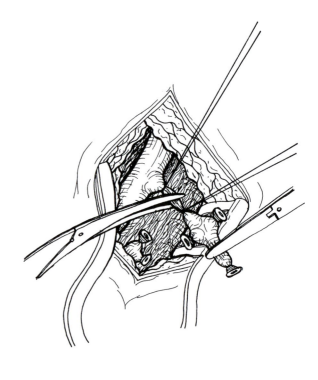

Fig. 18-6. Flush ligation of GSV at its origin from the common femoral vein.

■ POSTOPERATIVE INSTRUCTIONS

The patient is sent home with the pressure dressing in place and told that ambulation is permitted and recommended. If swelling occurs, the instructions are to elevate the extremity first and change the pressure dressing if necessary to relieve undue pain or swelling. If there is a problem with pain or swelling, it is better to check the wounds and dressings in the first 24 hours to rule out a bleed or other mishap in the procedure. A mild pain medication is prescribed for all patients, but most report that it either was not needed or wasn't used after the first evening.

The patient returns for an initial dressing on the first or second postoperative day. Of major importance is to explain to the patient the value of retaining effective compression for the remainder of the postoperative course and to reapply the dressing with their participation and understanding.

The duration of pressure in the postoperative period is an unsolved question. In the warmth of Hawaii patients are reluctant to keep a dressing in place for any length of time and even reluctant to wear a support

stocking. For this reason, we have experimented with short durations of support because it would be impossible to gain compliance with support for periods that approach six weeks. By trial and error, we have found precise support to be very necessary during the first week. Without this, there will be too many occurrences of hematomas both inside and outside the varices and too much hemosiderin staining. During the second and third weeks, we have found good results with fitted knee-length surgical compression stockings of 30 to 40 mm compression as an alternative to a large compression dressing. By the end of two to three weeks, most patients prefer to be out of support and find the cosmetic result adequate to go without dressings. Late hematomas developing after two weeks of compression are very rare, so we use this as a practical cut-off point in uncomplicated cases. When ulcers or lipodermatosclerosis are present, a long period of support is obviously indicated.

■ CLINICAL EXPERIENCE

During the latter half of the 1980s saphenofemoral ligation and sclerotherapy was advocated as the treatment of choice in our practice for most patients with varicose veins and incompetent GSVs; 80 to 100 of

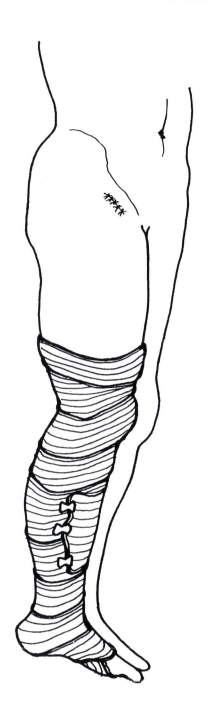

Fig. 18-7.   Completed operation and bandaged extremity ready for ambulation.

these procedures were performed each year. This policy was based upon a combination of factors that included a degree of dissatisfaction with the "radical" vein stripping of the classical Mayo technique,[11] a few instances of particularly vexsome saphenous nerve injuries, and an effort to devise a simpler and more cost-effective method of dealing with a large population of varicose-

vein patients. The evolution of this approach was described in the literature in our 1986 report[12] where factors of cost, patient satisfaction, and posttreatment complications were compared for sclerotherapy alone, saphenofemoral ligation with sclerotherapy, and saphenofemoral ligation with stripping by the "radical" technique. The findings in that report were that the ligation and sclerotherapy patients were well satisfied, the costs were considerably less than for vein stripping, and sclerotherapy of the varices alone was not appropriate for patients with incompetent GSV valves. This economic aspect was also reported by Neglen.[13]

With the passage of time following ligation and sclerotherapy, we found some patients returning with recurrent varices of significant proportions. They were nearly all found to have patent and incompetent saphenous veins that were fed either by neovascularization of the GSV at the proximal end or by thigh perforators; of these, neovascularization has been a much more frequent finding. When they were explored at surgery, the usual finding was a syncytium of tiny vessels in the scar of the ligation; these vessels communicated with the lumen of the retained GSV and produced recurrent proximal incompetence, which over time resulted in recurrent varicose veins. Rarely was a large missed vessel in the region of the saphenofemoral junction encountered that could explain the recurrence. This tendency of neovascularization in the venous system is also found in some patients after ligation and division of the superficial femoral vein. It appears to represent a physiologic response in the venous system at the femoral level. Although the frequency of clinically significant recurrence is not known in our experience, it is important to recognize this late-onset recurrence is a shortcoming of the ligation and sclerotherapy approach to varicose veins.

Although it is tempting to recall our patients to study their long-term results following ligation and sclerotherapy, it is unlikely we will learn anything that is not already obvious in the literature. It is well established by Hobbs' studies that recurrences are significantly less frequent in late follow-up after vein stripping than after lesser procedures.[6] In a prospective series from Sweden[14] clinical and physiologic data is detailed with the same conclusion and similar results to those reported by Hobbs. These studies should suffice to establish the point.

Of more value would be the development of a technique that would eliminate the neovascularization process. Perhaps a longer resection of the GSV in the thigh or obliteration of the upper ligated GSV with sclerosant will make a difference. There is a report from Australia of dissecting the pectineal fascia and sewing this over the proximal stump of the GSV.[15] Bergan advocates dissection of the divided tributaries beyond their first or even second bifurcation with avulsion of the vein beyond that point to minimize neovascularization.[8]

While new developments are awaited, there are reasons and times when the simpler procedure of ligation with sclerotherapy may be chosen over ligation with stripping, giving support to the concept of following a selective use of various procedures tailored to the clinical setting posed by the individual patient.

SELECTIVE INDICATIONS FOR TREATMENT

For the individual who mainly desires the veins to be eradicated once and forever, the best chance lies in the saphenofemoral ligation with stripping of the GSV. This is safely done on an outpatient basis and is relatively painless when done with good compression support postoperatively. By employing the alternative of stripping to the upper calf and using cosmetic stab-avulsion techniques for removing varices, the results are cosmetically excellent, and the time away from work is minimized compared with the grosser methods of stripping that were practiced in the past.

In other patients, the accent on recurrence is less than the desire to eliminate the mass of varices in a simple way. This is often true of the older aged patient who is more sedentary, but is still bothered by large varices or by superficial phlebitis in the varices, or of the younger patient who wants to preserve the GSV as a spare part. Those with a strong history of vascular disease in the family or the diabetic who may be more likely to need all of the potential spare parts may wish to save the GSV. Some patients, particularly males with a busy lifestyle and a low level of concern for small recurrent varicosities, may prefer a simpler procedure.

In the patient with complications of the axial (GSV) incompetence, such as lipodermatosclerosis or ulceration, stripping the GSV is preferred to avoid recurrence of these severe manifestations of the superficial incompetence.

These clinical variances led us to adopt a selective approach to treatment that is broadly outlined in the accompanying algorithm. A Doppler examination is a routine part of the physical in the office. For those who have no reflux in the GSV, sclerotherapy or stab phlebectomy is used to treat the varices without further testing. For those with GSV reflux, a duplex scan is used to separate patients with pure superficial saphenous incompetence from patients with accompanying deep-vein disease. When deep-vein involvement is found, further evaluation is often indicated. In patients with pure superficial saphenous incompetence, various considerations, such as age, activity level, presence of ulceration, family history of vascular disease, and patient preferences are used to decide between sclerotherapy and stripping with stab phlebectomy.

REFERENCES

1. Jacobsen BH: The value of different forms of treatment for varicose veins, Br J Surg 66:182-184, 1979.
2. Sladen JG: Flush ligation and compression sclerotherapy for the control of venous disease, Am J Surg, 152: 535-538, 1986.
3. Friedell ML, et al.: High ligation of the greater saphenous vein for treatment of lower extremity varicosities: the fate of the vein and therapeutic results, Ann Vasc Surg, 6:5-8, 1992.
4. Hammersten J, et al.: Long saphenous vein saving surgery for varicose veins. A long-term follow-up, Eur J Vasc Surg, 4:361-364, 1990.
5. Rutherford RB, Sawyer JD, Jones DN: The fate of residual saphenous vein after partial removal or ligation, J Vasc Surg, 12:422-428, 1990.
6. Hobbs JT: Surgery and sclerotherapy in the treatment of varicose veins, Arch Surg, 109:793-796, 1974.
7. Neglen P, Einarsson E, Eklof B: The functional long-term value of different types of treatment for saphenous vein incompetence, J Cardiovasc Surg, 34:295-301, 1993.
8. Bergan JJ: Surgical procedures for varicose veins: axial stripping and stab avulsion. In JJ Bergan, Kistner RL, editors: Atlas of venous surgery, Philadelphia, 1992, pp 61-75 W.B. Saunders Co.
9. Goldman MP: Mechanism of action of sclerotherapy. In MP Goldman, editor: Sclerotherapy: treatment of varicose and telangiectatic leg veins, St Louis, 1991, pp 183-191 Mosby Year Book.
10. Malouf GM, Conrad P: The Australian polidocanol (Aethoxysklerol) open clinical trial results at two years, presented at the American Venous Forum, 6th Annual Meeting, Maui, Hawaii, Feb. 24, 1994.
11. Lofgren KA: Management of varicose veins: the Mayo Clinic experience. In JJ Bergan, JST Yao, editors: Venous Problems, Chicago, 1978, pp 71-83 Year Book Medical.
12. Kistner RL, et al.: The evolving management of varicose veins: Straub Clinic experience, Postgraduate Medicine, 80:51-59, 1986.
13. Neglen P: Economical aspects of treatment of varicose veins. In Eklof B, Gjores JE, Thulesius O, Bergqvist D, editors, Controversies in the management of venous disorders, London: 1989, pp 234-239 Butterworths.
14. Neglen P, Einarsson E, Eklof B: High tie with sclerotherapy for saphenous vein insufficiency, Phlebology, 1: 105-111, 1980.
15. Sheppard M: A procedure for the prevention of recurrent saphenofemoral incompetence, Aust N Z J Surg 48: 322-326, 1978.

19

Recurrent Varicose Veins

Simon G. Darke

Superficial varicosities are known to affect between 10 and 12% of the adult population[1,2] with a familial tendency.[3] The recurrence rate after surgery, defined as patients seeking further advice and possible treatment, is formidable: It occurs in 20 to 30% of reported series whether assessed systematically at follow-up or in patients rereferred de novo for new appraisal.[4-12] These results are disappointing for both surgeons and patients and have important resource implications. Contemporary strategies in primary treatment, and improved diagnostic facilities and awareness, may have reduced this incidence.[12-15]

To maximize the effect of primary treatment and to rationalize management when recurrence does occur, it is of value to explore the underlying morphology of recurrence. Duplex scanning has become increasingly effective in this respect and is particularly valuable in view of its noninvasive nature. Furthermore the information gained has a practical value that can be used to illustrate by marking the patient immediately prior to surgery and by accompanying diagrams. This modality, however, is less useful in producing a descriptive and illustrative guide, as required in this book. Reliance here, therefore, has been placed on suitable venograms.

■ EVALUATION

History

In general, patients with recurrent varicose veins seeking advice are concerned either about cosmetic aspects or want reassurances about future implications of their condition. Excessive pain, swelling, or skin change denote more serious and complex problems.

This can be either primary deep incompetence or the consequences of previous deep-vein thrombosis.[12-15] In the context of what is considered here, it is essential that the latter is recognized. A careful enquiry should be made into any history of previous deep-vein thrombosis. This, however, is not always evident and cannot be relied upon to exclude the possibility. In half of those cases with venographic evidence of previous thrombosis, no patient awareness of such an incident exists.[16] Careful note should be made of the timing and nature of previous surgery. Sometimes these may have been repeated.[12] This fact and a strong familial history of varicose veins suggest that further recurrence is possible. Patients should be counseled and advised accordingly. This does not, in the authors view however, contraindicate further surgery even if the benefits may be of only medium-term duration.

Examination

The examination begins with the distribution of superficial varicosities (see Fig. 19-1). Previous scars should be noted. The value of the hand held doppler scanner, as with all varicose veins, cannot be over emphasized and should form an integral part of this initial examination. Of specific importance is to explore the possibility of incompetence in a second saphenous system (usually the saphenopopliteal, see later in this chapter). The techniques involved are outside the scope of this chapter, but have been described in detail elsewhere.[17]

Recurrent saphenofemoral incompetence is particularly significant and is suspected if there is a reflux signal over distal varicosities on patient coughing. This is an important sign that requires more detailed investigation because it implies an incompetent communication with the deep system.[12]

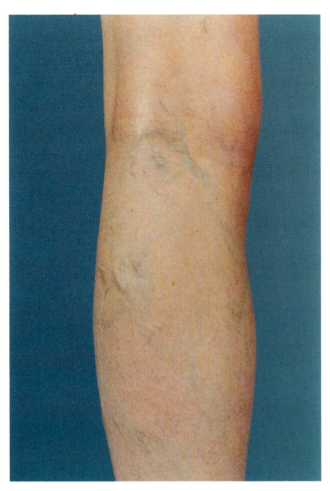

Fig. 19-1. A faint scar is evidence of previous saphenopopliteal exploration. Color duplex scanning reveals further problems arising from the medial gastrocnemius vein that feeds recurrent varicosities. This is treated by further exploration and ligation of the gastrocnemius vein under general anesthetic and hook avulsions of superficial varicosities. Co-existent reticular and telangiectatic veins are treated subsequently with compression sclerotherapy.

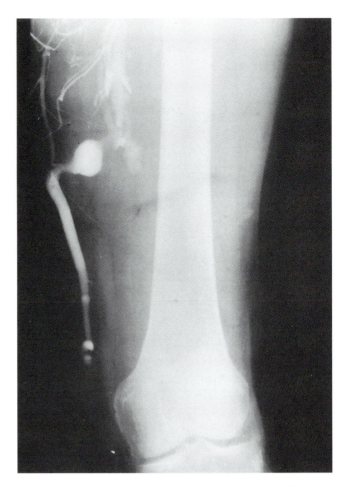

Fig. 19-2. Type 1 recurrence. Ascending venogram shows an incompetent thigh perforator feeding a persistent, long, saphenous trunk. Treated by accurate preoperative duplex localization, ligation of perforator and closure of deep-fascial defect; excision of residual, long saphenous trunk from knee area to point of entry.

▪ INVESTIGATIONS

Venography

Reference has already been made to the need to exclude previous deep-vein thrombosis. In this respect, ascending venography remains the most sensitive. With suitable tourniquets, this is also the means by which incompetent calf and thigh perforators can be demonstrated (see Fig. 19-2).[16] Descending venograms will demonstrate the nature of recurrent saphenofemoral reflux (see illustrations) and the presence of primary deep incompetence (see illustrations). In some instances incompetent thigh perforating veins and recurrent saphenopopliteal reflux can be demonstrated (see illustrations).[12,16] Varicography can be useful in demonstrating the communication of superficial varicosities with the deep system.[18]

Duplex

Reference has already been made to duplex, particularly color, as an invaluable tool both in determining the underlying morphology and mapping veins immediately prior to surgery. It is outside the scope of this chapter to expand this modality, but it is particularly valuable in the saphenopopliteal area, which has wide anatomical variations and complex incompetent venous origins.[19]

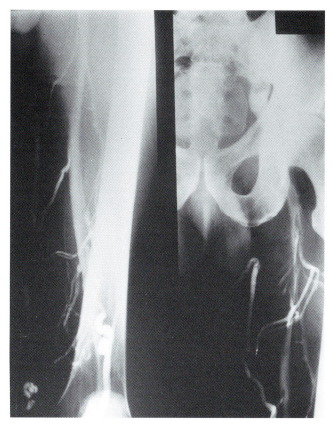

Fig. 19-3. Type 1 recurrence through multiple small thigh perforators. It is often impractical in this complex situation to identify and ligate all these sources of origin. A pragmatic compromise might consist of either local superficial avulsions or compression sclerotherapy and recognition that further recurrences may occur in a few years' time.

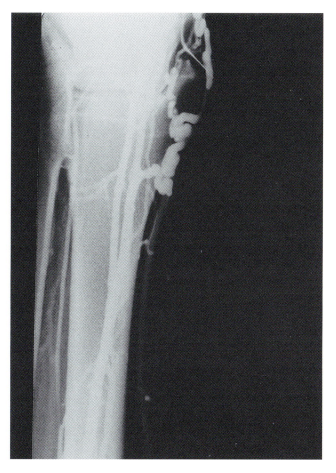

Fig. 19-4. Type 1 recurrence through an ankle perforator, isolated to the calf. This is uncommon. Treated by accurate preoperative localization with duplex, ligation, and closure of fascial defect in a similar fashion as described in Fig. 19-2.

Quantified Test of Venous Function

It is outside the scope of this chapter to consider these in detail. However, a variety of modalities, principally plethysmographic, are available to evaluate the venous outflow. In recurrent varicose veins this is important when concerns about previous deep-vein thrombosis exist. It can be applied specifically to determine the functional role of superficial varicosities. A compromise in venous outflow with the application of appropriate tourniquets can indicate these to be important and functional collaterals. Intervention under these circumstances is contraindicated.

Patterns of Recurrence

To establish the frequency and underlying morphology of recurrence I have evaluated the findings in 444 patients referred consecutively to me.[12] This is to a secondary referral center from a relatively captive population. It is therefore thought to be a relatively pure and representative sample of the problem as it exists.

Of these patients, 95 (21%) had had previous surgery confirmed by history and by the presence of scars in appropriate areas sited at either the saphenofemoral or the saphenopopliteal junction. All these patients had concerns or symptoms of sufficient import to be seeking advice regarding further surgery. Clinical examination, ultrasound including hand-held doppler and duplex, and ascending and descending venography in appropriate cases were used to evaluate those patients. By these means patients were categorized into one of three different types.

Type 1: No evidence of recurrent incompetence of either saphenofemoral or saphenopopliteal junctions. Varicography in these patients revealed that the source is either through thigh or calf perforating vein(s) or both.

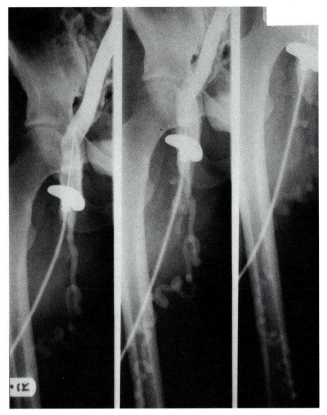

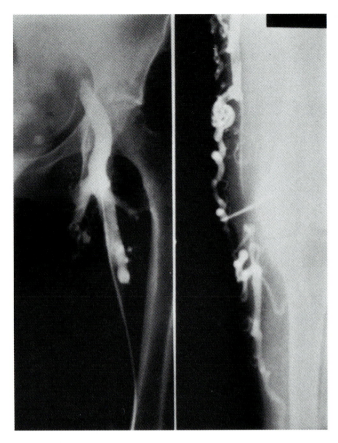

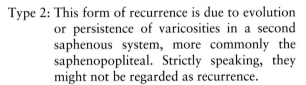

Fig. 19-5. Type 3A recurrence. Recurrent saphenofemoral reflux caused by an untied tributary at the time of original surgery. Treated by further flush ligation.

Fig. 19-6. Type 3A recurrence. In this instance the main trunk of the saphenofemoral junction was missed during the original surgery because the previous approach was too low. Treated by accurate ligation and multiple avulsions.

Type 2: This form of recurrence is due to evolution or persistence of varicosities in a second saphenous system, more commonly the saphenopopliteal. Strictly speaking, they might not be regarded as recurrence.

Type 3: These patients are the most complex and are demonstrated by hand-held doppler scanners to have a positive cough impulse in a distal varicosity (see earlier). This is evidence of an incompetent communication(s) with the deep system. These patients can be further divided into three subcategories:

3A: An untied tributary at the groin caused by inadequate or incomplete surgery at the time of the original operation.

3B: Incompetence in the superficial femoral vein and a thigh perforator (these could be regarded as Type 1).

3C: Reconstruction of the saphenofemoral junction caused by the process of neovascularization.[12]

Table 19-1 Type of recurrence

Total recurrences		95
Type 1	Thigh perforator	29
Type 2	Emergence of SPI	9
	Emergence of SFI	1
Type 3	Recurrent SFI	46
	Recurrent SPI	10

Table 19-2

Total number limbs evaluated		47
3A	United tributary	4
3B	Incompetent SFV and thigh perforator	9
3C	Reconstituted junction	28
3B & 3C	Combined	4

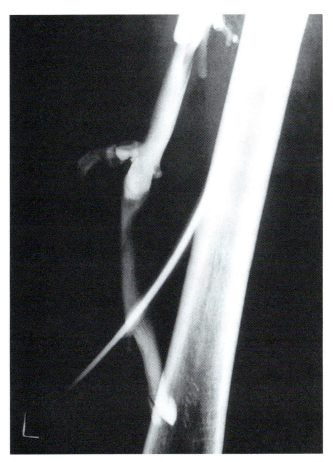

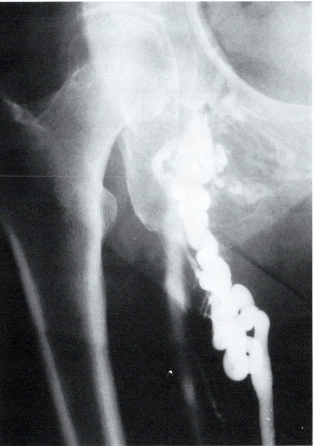

A

Fig. 19-7. Type 3B recurrent saphenofemoral incompetence. A positive cough impulse will be heard on the distally situated varicosities with a hand-held doppler scanner. This descending venogram shows reflux down the superficial femoral vein and out through an incompetent thigh perforator. Treated by accurate preoperative duplex localization and local ligation. Deep incompetence remains a problem in this situation and can contribute to further recurrence. Vein-valve repair, however, should only be considered if coexistent ulceration exists.

Fig. 19-8. **A** and **B**, examples of Type 3C recurrence caused by reconstitution of the saphenofemoral junction by neovascularization. The typical complex multichanneled appearance is reconnecting the persistent, long, saphenous trunk with the common femoral vein. Treated by reexploration and accurate religation at the points of origin from the common femoral vein. Coverage of the denuded common femoral vein can be augmented by using a rotated strip of fascia lata or applying a Dacron patch. Excision of the residual, long, saphenous trunk from knee level is advisable.

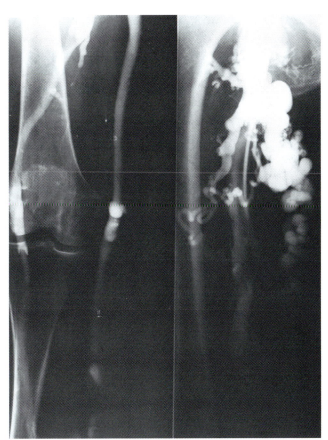

B

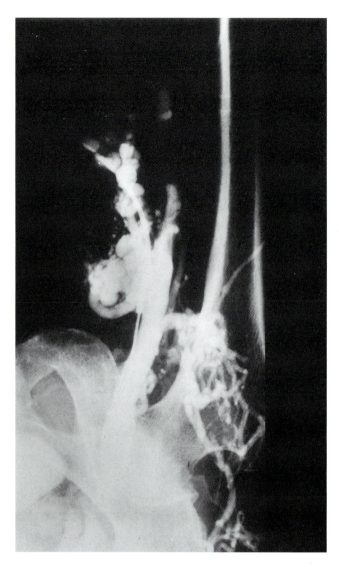

Fig. 19-9. Type 3C recurrence due to reconstitution. In this instance there is no persistent, long, saphenous trunk. This illustrates that this phenomenon can occur even when adequate saphenous excision has been previously undertaken. Treated by flush ligation.

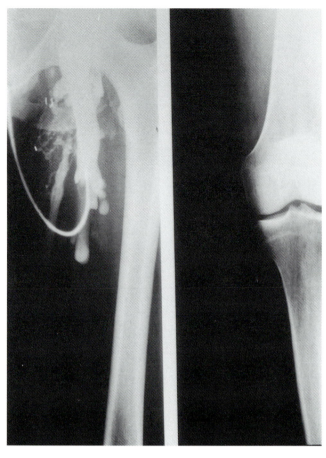

Fig. 19-10. Descending venogram showing the very early phases and rapid evolution of neovascularization and the development of Type 3C recurrence. This was taken only five months after previous groin ligation under local anesthetic with retention of incompetent, long, saphenous trunk at another institute. The patient already displayed extensive recurrent and persistent varicosities with a cough impulse through these minor channels. It illustrates that in those individuals idiosyncratically predisposed; simple groin ligation alone, without saphenous trunk excision, carries a significant risk of recurrence of this nature.

A few patients had more than one form.

The relative frequency of these forms of recurrence are shown in Tables 19-1 and 19-2. Rarely recurrence can occur through obturator, ovarian, round ligament, and deep-femoral veins (see illustrations).

■ Treatment

The underlying principle in treating recurrent varicose veins is to secure, whenever reasonably possible, the connecting origin from the deep-venous system.

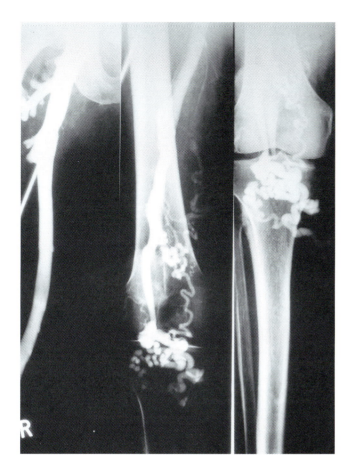

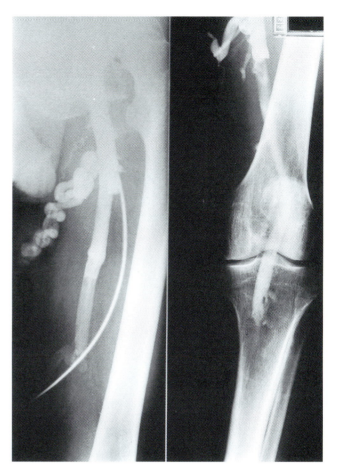

Fig. 19-11. A descending venogram in a patient with an incompetent femoropopliteal segment, thus fortuitously allowing the imaging of a recurrent saphenopopliteal junction. This is strikingly similar to the appearance seen in Fig. 20-8 and 20-9 and caused by reconstitution by neovascularization (Type 3C). Reexploration under these circumstances is difficult and potentially hazardous and should always be preceded by accurate preoperative duplex mapping.

Fig. 19-12. Complex dual recurrence through a Type 3C reconstituted saphenofemoral junction and incompetent thigh veins.

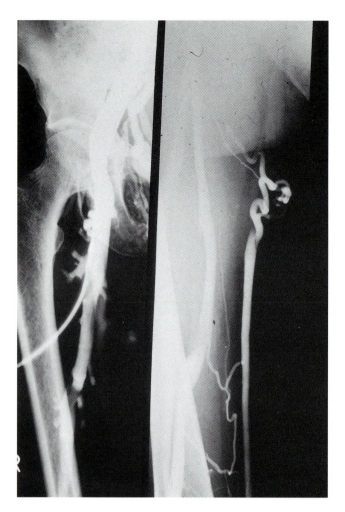

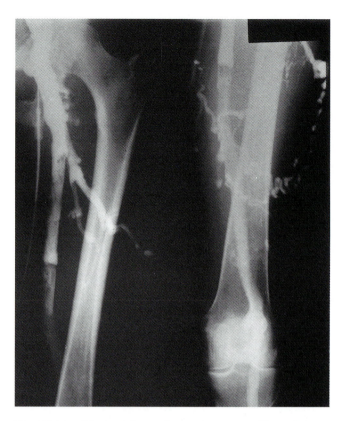

Fig. 19-14. Unusual form of recurrence caused by reflux down an incompetent, deep-femoral vein and out through a distal communication with the posterior thigh vein. Treated by superficial avulsions only or compression sclerotherapy.

Fig. 19-13. Complex recurrence occurring through both pelvic veins feeding a persistent long saphenous trunk. Treated by the excision of the persistent trunk and multiple phlebotomies only. This type of recurrence is likely to pose future problems, and the patient should be warned accordingly.

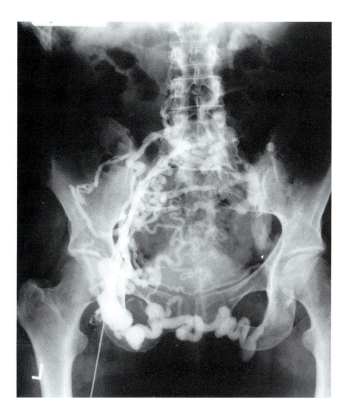

Fig. 19-15. Patient with massive recurrent pubic varicosities caused by extensive previous and unknown vena caval and iliac thrombosis. Surgical intervention strongly contraindicated.

■ REFERENCES

1. Coon WW, Willis PW III, Keller JB: Venous thromboembolism and other venous disease in the Tecumseh Community Health Study, Circulation 48:839-850, 1973.

2. Widmer LK, Mall T, Martin H: Epidemiology and sociomedical importance of peripheral venous disease. In Jobbs JT, editor: The treatment of venous disorders, Lancaster, 1977, pp 3-12, MTP Press Ltd.

3. Reagan B, Folse R: Lower limb haemodynamics in normal persons and children of patients with varicose veins, Surg Gynaecol Obstet 132:15-22, 1971.

4. Hobbs JT: Surgery and sclerotherapy in the treatment of varicose veins, Arch Surg 109:793-796, 1974.

5. Doran FSA, White M: A clinical trial to discover if primary treatment of varicose veins should be by Fagan's method or by an operation, Br J Surgery 62:72-6, 1975.

6. Sheppard M: A procedure for the prevention of recurrent sapheno femoral incompetence, Aust NZ J Surgery 48:322-326, 1978.

7. Jakobsen BH: The value of different forms of treatment for varicose veins, Br J Surgery 66:182-184, 1979.

8. Lofgren EP: Treatment of long saphenous varicosities and their recurrence: a long-term follow up. In Bergan JJ, Yao JST, editors: Surgery of the veins, Orlando, 1985, Grune & Stratton.

9. Royle JP: Recurrent varicose veins, World of Surgery 10:944-953, 1986.

10. Beridge DC, Makin GS: Day case surgery; a viable alternative for surgical treatment of varicose veins, Phlebology 2:103-108, 1987.

11. Einarrson E, Eklof B, Norgren L: Compression sclerotherapy or operation for primary varicose veins. In Proceedings of VII Int. Cong. of Phlebography, Copenhagen 1.

12. Darke SG: The morphology of recurrent varicose veins, European J Vascular Surgery 6:512-517, 1992.

13. Darke SG: Chronic venous insufficiency—should the long saphenous vein be stripped? In Barros D'Sa AAB, Bell PRF, Darke SG, Harris PL: Vascular surgery current questions, Oxford, 1991, pp 207-218, Butterworth-Hennemann.

14. Darke SG: Surgical management of superficial vein problems. In Yao JST, Pearce WH: Long term results in vascular surgery, Norwalk, Conn., 1993, pp 411-426, Appleton & Longe.

15. Darke SG: Varicose veins. In Galland RB, Clyne CAC: Clinical problems in vascular surgery, London, 1994, pp 215-221, Edward Arnold.

16. Darke SG, Andress MR: The value of venography in the management of chronic venous disorders of the lower limb. In Greenhalgh RM, editor: Diagnostic techniques and assessment procedures in vascular surgery, Orlando, 1985, pp 421-446, Grune & Stratton.

17. Mitchell DC, Darke SG: The assessment of primary varicose veins by Doppler ultrasound—the role of sapheno popliteal incompetence and the short saphenous system in calf varicosities. European J vascular surgery 1:113-115, 1987.

18. Corbett CR, McIrvine AJ, Aston NO, Jamieson CW, Lea Thomas ML: The use of varicography to identify the sources of incompetence in recurrent varicose veins, Annals Royal College of Surgeons 66:412-415, 1982.

19. Darke SG: Recurrent varicose veins and short saphenous insufficiency. In Bergan JJ, Jao JST: Venous disorders, Philadelphia, 1991, pp 217-232, W.B. Saunders Co.

20

Endoscopic Subfascial Perforator Vein Interruption

John J. Bergan

At the end of the 1930s, Robert Linton of Boston emphasized the need for control of perforating veins in treatment of chronic, recurrent, venous ulceration.[1] Reports of this procedure's use during the next 30 years suggested that it succeeded for the most part.[2] However, recurrence of ulcerations 5 and 10 years after surgery dimmed enthusiasm for the operation.[3] Further, the long hospitalization times required by the slow secondary healing of long incisions from the retromalleolar ankle to knee discouraged wide application of the operation.[4]

Perforator vein interruption was virtually the only available surgical procedure and was effective in 60 to 85% of patients operated upon.[5] Therefore, numerous variations were advocated.[6] All of these required inpatient hospitalization and variable immobility time to heal surgical incisions and associated ulcerations.

Introduction of laparoscopic general surgery spurred investigation of minimally invasive approaches to venous surgery. Accumulating experience suggested that video-assisted techniques might be applicable to subfascial perforator interruption because 90% of incompetent perforating veins occur in the lower leg in the posterior arch vein distribution.[7]

Clinically significant perforators include the gastrocnemius point, soleal point, and perforating veins identified at varying distances from the heel pad.[8] All of these are accessible by endoscopic coagulation or clipping. Such interruption occludes the perforating vein proximal to its branchings, and this approach allows transection of all perforators that are thought to be significant clinically. An appealing aspect of the procedure is that it can be performed on an outpatient basis. Further, the surgical incision is made proximal to affected skin even in patients with far-advanced changes of lipodermatosclerosis and healed ulceration.

Conrad, in Australia, and Gloviczki, at the Mayo Clinic, use gas insufflation techniques as used in laparoscopic surgery. These create a widely subfascial space through which perforator interruption can be accomplished easily. However, maintaining gas pressure is difficult. The fascial seal is frequently interrupted by scope manipulation.

O'Donnell uses physiologic liquid distention of the subfascial space with irrigation of the area to be explored.[9] He believes that Ringer's lactate solution infused through the subfascial space is safer than using CO_2, which might penetrate the venous system.

We have chosen to modify the open technique of Reinhard Fischer of St. Gallen, Switzerland.[10]

■ Incision

The incision is made on the anteromedial leg posterior to the tibia. The 3 cm skin and subcutaneous incision is retracted to expose the fascia, which is incised. A subfascial space is created by inserting the endoscope and manipulating it anteriorly as far as is feasible and then posteriorly as far as needed.

It is relatively easy to distinguish a normal perforating vein that is competent from one that is incompetent. The normal perforator exhibits one or more veins with parallel walls that are not tortuous or dilated. The accompanying artery is often seen. In contrast, the incompetent perforating vein is often thick, passes transversely, is apparently white and looks bloodless if a tourniquet is used and limb exsanguination has preceded the exploration. Without the tourniquet the incompetent perforating vein looks like any other varicose vein. Frequently, the incompetent perforating vein branches into one or more tributaries before penetrating the fascia. Recognition of perforating veins is much more accurate by the subfascial approach than by phlebography or preoperative Doppler or duplex technique.

Limitations of subfascial video endoscopic perforator interruption are found in the most distal aspect of the leg. This is a dangerous area anatomically. Here, there is reduced maneuverability of the instrumentation. The most serious distal consequences of the procedure include posterior tibial nerve damage. Complications can be avoided by keeping strictly to the fascia in every step throughout the endoscopy. Also, no structure should be divided unless one is absolutely sure it is a perforating vein. Before applying the cautery, extreme care must be taken that the structure being clamped, cauterized, or clipped is a perforating vein and not the accompanying artery or posterior tibial nerve.

ALTERNATIVE TECHNIQUES

The blind subfascial perforator interruption popularized by Hach[11] has been widely used. DePalma has advocated a variation of this.[12] However, with these blind methods, there is no way to be sure that perforating veins have been divided. The paratibial perforating veins, which are also very important, cannot be severed using this technique.

HISTORIC DEVELOPMENT

Subfascial endoscopy-assisted perforator interruption initially began using available instruments such as the mediastinoscope. Instruments were already in use and were familiar. The technique proved to be as simple as looking through a mediastinoscope, identifying the perforating vein, and dividing it. However, as Fischer said, ". . . at times it is a bit troublesome for the back of the surgeon." Fischer also called attention to the fact that at times it is somewhat difficult to distinguish the accompanying nerve.[13]

Hauer[14] introduced the angulated scope and its offset, fiberoptic, lighting and video camera that provided magnification and better examination of anatomic details. The original instruments advocated by Hauer were expensive and imperfect to manipulate.

Gerhard Sattler[15] subsequently refined the instrumentation with the help of the Storz instrument company. The angulated optics allow mounting of the video camera at a 45-degree angle, thus providing an 11-mm working channel to be used with a 30-cm scope. With this, anatomic details are more easily recognized, and the accompanying nerves can be separated from the perforating veins. The procedure's cost has been markedly reduced because of adaptability of the particular instruments to available video monitors.

Bradbury and Ruckley[16] of Edinburgh have identified those patients who might fail the subfascial perforator interruption. They studied 53 patients who had standard, open, subfascial ligation of perforating veins with saphenous ligation. All operations were done for recurrent venous ulcerations, and studies performed preoperatively and postoperatively were remarkably complete. Patients with popliteal venous incompetence were found to have reduced, venous-expulsion fraction and refill times as venous ulcers recurred. Patients can, therefore, be selected for subfascial perforator interruption on the basis of duplex studies that demonstrate deep-venous competence distal to the superficial femoral vein.

FASCIOTOMY

Division of the crural fascia in patients with the most severe forms of chronic venous insufficiency has been advocated by many.[17] The subfascial endoscopic perforator interruption technique lends itself to such fasciotomy. After division of the perforating veins and thorough exploration of the available space, the procedure is terminated by passing a fasciotomy knife through the scope and incising the fascia from above downward or from below upward. The pathophysiologic indication for this is the changes observed in the fascia in severe, chronic, venous insufficiency. Thickening and induration so regularly found are thought to limit transfascial blood flow. Subfascial compartment pressures are elevated in patients with severe forms of chronic venous insufficiency. These compartmental pressures fall after fasciotomy and remain at a lower level over prolonged periods of observation.

Modern methods of fasciotomy have been introduced by Hach[14] and updated, including a paratibial approach by Vanscheidt.[16] Postoperative magnetic resonance studies performed at three and six months after fasciotomy have shown that the broad fasciotomy split is still visible at least six months following the procedure.

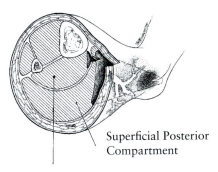

Superficial Posterior
Compartment

Deep Posterior Compartment

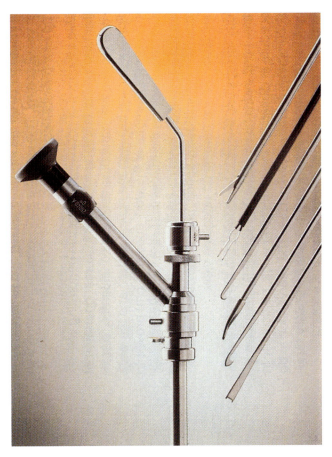

Fig. 20-1. This artist's drawing shows the placement of the skin, subcutaneous, and fascial incisions that allow the physician access to the posterior compartment of the leg. Space is created by manipulating the endoscope, and the technique is performed without gas or liquid insufflation. Paratibial perforating veins are approached through an additional fascial incision into the deep posterior compartment, as indicated in this diagram.

Fig. 20-3. It is the Storz endoscopic instrumentation modified by Sattler that has proved most useful in subfascial endoscopic techniques. Modifications of the dissection instrumentation of Reinhard Fischer are also shown in this photograph. These instruments are used to mobilize the vessels to separate nerves and arteries from perforating veins. The prograde and retrograde knives used for fasciotomy are also illustrated.

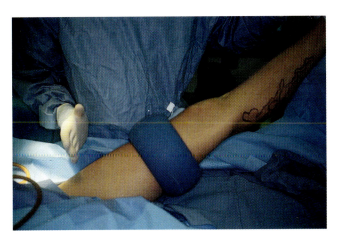

Fig. 20-2. A proximal thigh tourniquet considerably eases performance of the subfascial video-assisted perforator interruption. Although the Lofqvist tourniquet is shown here, in America the use of an Esmarch bandage to exsanguinate the leg before inflating an orthopedic tourniquet has proved eminently satisfactory.

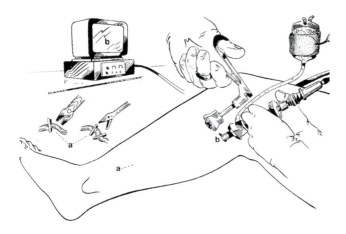

Fig. 20-4. O'Donnell has pioneered use of the subfascial perforator interruption technique in this country. His technique of Ringer's lactate irrigation of the subfascial space and use of two ports is illustrated here. Procedure techniques are still under investigation, and modifications of current technology will be inevitable. (from Bergan JJ, Kistner RL: Atlas of venous surgery, Philadelphia, 1992, W.B. Saunders Co., with permission).

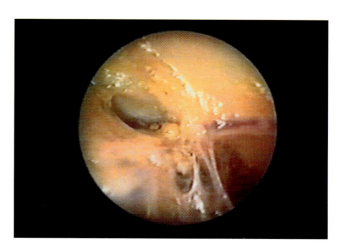

Fig. 20-6. Perforating veins and their accompanying arteries are identified under the magnification of the scope, and clean dissection is possible. (Courtesy Gerhard Sattler, Darmstadt.)

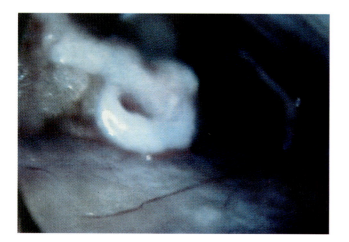

Fig. 20-5. Perforating veins are seen as large, tortuous, white structures in the subfascial space. In this operative photograph, the fascia is seen superiorly, and the perforating vein is identified by its white, glistening, dilated appearance.

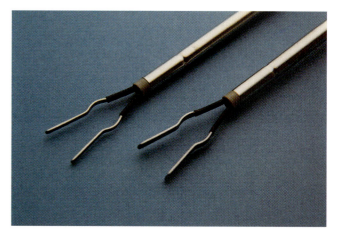

Fig. 20-7. The 1 and 2 mm electrocoagulation instruments allow hemostasis to be achieved before division of the perforating vein. (Courtesy Gerhard Sattler, Darmstadt.)

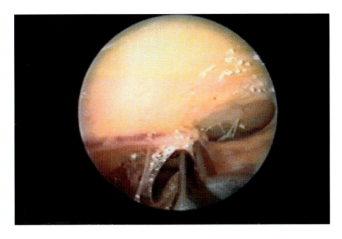

Fig. 20-8. This figure shows the electrocoagulation instrument in place on the perforating vein just as electric current is applied to the tips of the coagulation clamps. (Courtesy Gerhard Sattler, Darmstadt.)

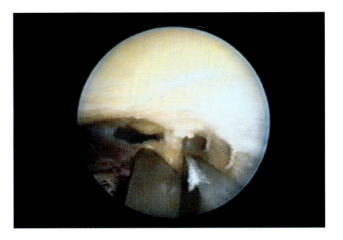

Fig. 20-10. The perforating vein is shown being cut by the angulated scissor in this photograph. (Courtesy Gerhard Sattler, Darmstadt.)

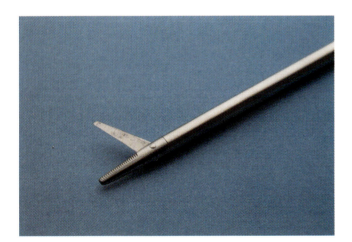

Fig. 20-9. The angulated, serrated scissor, adaptable to the 11 mm working channel of the scope, permits division of the perforating vein. (Courtesy Gerhard Sattler, Darmstadt.)

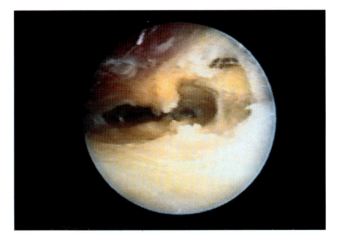

Fig. 20-11. Clean division of the perforating vein without bleeding is achieved by electrocoagulation followed by transection. The stump of the vein can be seen entering the fascia superiorly and the residual origin of the perforator is retracted towards the inferiorly located flexor muscle. (Courtesy Gerhard Sattler, Darmstadt.)

■ REFERENCES

1. Linton R: Communicating veins of the lower leg and the operative technique for their ligation, Ann Surg 107:582, 1938.

2. Silver D, Gleysteen JJ, Rhodes GR, et al.: Surgical treatment of the refractory postphlebitic ulcer, Arch Surg 103:554-460 1961.

3. Burnand KG, Lea Thomas M, O'Donnell T, Browse NL: Relation between postphlebitic changes in deep veins and results of treatment of venous ulcers, Lancet 1: 936-38, 1976.

4. Bowen FH: Subfascial ligation (Linton Operation) of the perforating leg veins to treat post-thrombophlebitic syndrome, American Surgeon 41:148-51, 1975.

5. Mayberry JC, Moneta GL, Taylor LM, Jr., Porter MJ: Nonoperative treatment of venous ulcer. In Bergan JJ, Yao JST, editors: Venous disorders, Philadelphia, 1991, pp 381-95, WB Saunders Co.

6. DePalma RG: Surgical therapy for venous stasis: results of a modified Linton operation, Am J Surg 137:810-13, 1979.

7. Jugenheimer M, Junginger TH: Endoscopic subfascial sectioning of incompetent perforating veins in treatment of primary varicosis, World J Surg 16:971-75, 1992.

8. Sherman RS: Varicose veins: anatomy, reevaluation of Trendelenburg tests, and operating procedure, Surg Clin North Am 44:1369, 1964.

9. O'Donnell TF: Surgical treatment of incompetent communicating veins. In Bergan JJ, Kistner RL, editors. Atlas of venous surgery. Philadelphia, 1992, W.B. Saunders.

10. Fischer R: Erfahrungen mit der endoskopischen Perforantensanierung, Phebologie 21:224-29, 1992.

11. Hach R, Vanderpuye R: Operationstechnik der paratibialen Fasziotomie, Med Welt 36:1616-18, 1985.

12. DePalma RG: Surgical treatment of chronic venous ulceration. In Bergan JJ, Yao JST, editors: Venous disorders, Philadelphia, 1991, Chapter 28, W.B. Saunders Co.

13. Fischer R, Fullemann H-J, Alder W: Zum phlebologischen dogma der pradilektionstellen der Cockettschen Venae perforantes, Phlebol u Proktol 16:184-7, 1987.

14. Hauer G, et al.: Endoskopische subfasziale diszision der Perforansvenen. In Brunner H (Hrsg): Der Unterschenkel: aktuelle Probleme in der Angiologie 44,S:187-92. Toronto, 1988, Huber, Bern, Stuttgart.

15. Sattler G, et al.: Weiterentwicklung der endoskopischen Perforantendiszision mit Hilfe ciner Stablinsenoptik, 31. Kongress der deutschen Gesellschaft für Phlebologie. Frankfurt, 1991.

16. Bradbury AW, Stonebridge PA, Callam MJ, Allan P, Ruckley CV: Foot volumetry and ultrasonography in patients with recurrent ulceration after superficial and perforating vein ligation, Br J Surg 80:846-48, 1993.

17. Vanscheidt W, Peschen M, Kreitinger J, Schopf E: Paratibial fasciotomy, Phlebology 23:45-48, 1994.

INDEX